LITHIUM

LITHIUM

A DOCTOR, A DRUG, AND A BREAKTHROUGH

Walter A. Brown

LIVERIGHT PUBLISHING CORPORATION
A Division of W. W. Norton & Company
Independent Publishers Since 1923

For information about permission to reproduce selections from this book, write to
Permissions, Liveright Publishing Corporation,
a division of W. W. Norton & Company, Inc.,
500 Fifth Avenue, New York, NY 10110

For information about special discounts for bulk purchases, please contact
W. W. Norton Special Sales at specialsales@wwnorton.com or 800-233-4830

Manufacturing by LSC Communications, Harrisonburg
Book design by Brooke Koven
Production manager: Anna Oler

Library of Congress Cataloging-in-Publication Data

Names: Brown, Walter Armin, author.
Title: Lithium : a doctor, a drug, and a breakthrough / Walter A. Brown.
Description: First edition. | New York : Liveright Publishing Corporation,
[2019] | Includes bibliographical references and index.
Identifiers: LCCN 2019004546 | ISBN 9781631491993 (hardcover)
Subjects: | MESH: Cade, J. F. J. | Lithium Compounds—history | Antimanic
Agents—history | Lithium Compounds—therapeutic use | Bipolar
Disorder—history | Bipolar Disorder—drug therapy | Antimanic
Agents—therapeutic use
Classification: LCC RC516 .B78 2019 | NLM QV 77.9 | DDC 616.89/5061—dc23
LC record available at https://lccn.loc.gov/2019004546

ISBN 978-1-63149-790-2 pbk.

Liveright Publishing Corporation, 500 Fifth Avenue, New York, N.Y. 10110
www.wwnorton.com

W. W. Norton & Company Ltd., 15 Carlisle Street, London W1D 3BS

1 2 3 4 5 6 7 8 9 0

CONTENTS

INTRODUCTION

In July of 1968, I arrived at Yale, a newly minted doctor eager to start my specialty training in psychiatry. Back then, Freud's theories still dominated the field, and Yale was a veritable bastion of psychoanalysis. But I didn't learn much about psychoanalysis that year. What I did learn was not to approach Mr. G without first removing my necktie.

For the whole of that first year, I worked on a locked hospital ward, a place that housed the most severely mentally ill, and Mr. G was my first patient. A cherubic-looking 36-year-old, Mr. G had spent most of the last 17 years of his life in psychiatric hospitals, either immobilized by suicidal depression or in the throes of manic excitement—elated, talking nonstop, constantly on the move, chock full of plans. When I took on his care, Mr. G had one big plan. He was going to Washington to meet with the president.

My job was to make sure that didn't happen.

Several times a week, Mr. G would make a rush for the door. Three nurses and I would drag him to a seclusion room where I would wrestle him to a mattress and a nurse would inject him with a sedative. That's when I learned not to approach Mr. G without first removing my necktie; it was the first thing he would grab.

Mr. G suffered from manic-depressive illness, now more commonly known as bipolar disorder. The illness was officially renamed in the 1980 edition of the American Psychiatric Association's diagnostic manual; the manual's authors felt that the term *bipolar* was both more specific and less stigmatizing, *manic* being suggestive of the pejorative "maniac." Recognized since the second century CE, bipolar disorder, with its frequent periods of depression and mania, is among the most devastating of psychiatric conditions. And Mr. G wasn't alone in his affliction. About 1 percent of the world population—including well over 2 million Americans—endure this illness.

On a bright Tuesday morning in late November, as I rode my bicycle to the entrance of the hospital, I spotted Mr. G running across the parking lot on his way to the train station. Leaping off my bike, I managed to intercept him and convince him to come back to the ward. But his days there were numbered. His escape convinced the staff that Mr. G needed to be confined to a long-term facility, so he was transferred to the state hospital.

Two years later, after completing a research fellowship at the National Institutes of Health, I resumed my psychiatry training. Soon after, I ran into Mr. G, this time in the waiting room of a psychiatry clinic. Mr. G. brought me up to date on his situation. More than a year ago he had been released from the state hospital. Now he was living on his own and working as an assistant manager at a supermarket. His erratic behavior, emergency room visits, and hospital confinements were things of the past. He spoke with a combination of amusement and embarrassment about his single-minded determination to meet the president. Mr. G went on to tell me that a month before he left the hospital, he had started taking a drug that had just become available: lithium.

Now, more than 40 years after seeing how profoundly lithium changed Mr. G, I continue to be fascinated by its power.

Lithium, a light metal, is widely distributed on earth, with large amounts in rocks and seawater. Like the closely related metals sodium and potassium, when ingested, lithium readily enters cells throughout the body and takes part in cellular metabolism and other basic biological processes. Lithium's ability to fully alleviate the symptoms of a devastating condition makes it one of the best treatments in medicine. As again and again I saw the relief that lithium brought to my patients, I grew increasingly interested in how it worked and, in particular, how its remarkable effects were discovered. Over the years I gathered scattered bits of information, and each successive piece of the puzzle raised more questions. The original paper describing lithium's beneficial effects in manic patients—written by an Australian psychiatrist named John Cade—came out in 1949, but the Food and Drug Administration (FDA) did not approve lithium for use until 1970. Why the 20-year hiatus? There was a general sense in the psychiatric community that lithium's discovery was a lucky accident, but was that true, or was a more systematic process at play? Most of all, I wanted to find out how an unknown Australian psychiatrist named John Cade managed to accomplish something so profound. Who was this man, and what were the circumstances that brought him to a groundbreaking moment?

I went in search of the story of John Cade and his remarkable discovery. A crucial experiment on guinea pigs prompted him to take lithium himself, and eventually he tested it in manic patients. Cade's life brought him to the point where—equipped with neither research training nor research funding, working from a makeshift laboratory in an unused kitchen on the grounds of a small, isolated mental asylum—he set out to find the cause of, and cure for, manic-depressive illness.

In Cade's day, the first half of the twentieth century, most doctors believed that people with a chronic severe mental illness had a disease that was largely hereditary and that involved a brain abnormality. Other than electroshock for depression, there were no effective treatments. The customary therapy for these patients was to confine them in asylums indefinitely or until the condition spontaneously improved. Drugs with stimulating or sedating properties, amphetamines, opiates, and bromides among them, were administered with little benefit and no effect on the characteristic symptoms of the illness. The idea that a drug alone could alleviate the symptoms of manic depression seemed far-fetched in the extreme.

Although psychopharmacology is now an indispensable feature of contemporary life, John Cade's lithium discovery represented a radical departure from the prevailing ideas about the treatment of mental illness. It was the first demonstration that a drug can alleviate the fundamental symptoms of a mental illness. As such, Cade's discovery launched psychiatry's pharmacological revolution—the use of drugs to treat the mentally ill. Within a decade, antipsychotic and antidepressant drugs, such as chlorpromazine and imipramine, were identified. These types of drugs, along with lithium, continue to be the mainstays of psychiatric treatment, and they have not been appreciably improved upon. Lithium, however, differs in an important way from the psychiatric drugs that came in its wake. The other drugs are nonspecific: they alleviate a broad range of symptoms in several disorders. For example, so-called antidepressants, like the infamous fluoxetine (Prozac), provide at least as much relief from anxiety as they do from depression; and the antipsychotic drugs, like olanzapine (Zyprexa) and risperidone (Risperdal), so vital to the treatment of schizophrenia, are also widely used to treat the agitation and hallucinations associated with dementia and are useful as well in treating depression and anxiety. Lithium, on the other hand, is uniquely specific: it is effective only in manic-depressive illness.

Following up on Cade's discovery, other researchers found that lithium not only alleviates mania but actually prevents future episodes of mania and depression. Now a standard treatment for bipolar disorder, lithium enables most people with this formerly devastating condition to lead normal lives. Because of lithium and a few drugs that have come in its wake, those who suffer from bipolar disorder are no longer periodically hospitalized in the throes of manic excitement or melancholic despair. Cade's break-through has prevented millions of suicides and salvaged an untold number of lives. It has also saved the world economy hundreds of billions of dollars in hospitalization costs. By 1994, 20 years after it was approved by the FDA to treat manic-depressive illness, lith-ium was estimated to have saved the U.S. economy $145 billion.[1]

Despite the inarguable significance of his discovery, Cade, the man, is little known outside of Australian psychiatric cir-cles. What is known about him from the testimony of colleagues, his family, and his own writings suggests, at first glance, that he was an unlikely candidate for scientific immortality. Some of his ideas about what causes mental illness—and what sorts of matters warranted investigation—could be charitably described as naive (at one point he was convinced that inadequate intake of fruit causes schizophrenia); and he had no formal research training. His research approach, by his own admission, was to putter about and see what turned up.

Equally unpromising was his work environment. Cade's labo-ratory, where he did the background research on lithium, was an abandoned kitchen on the grounds of a mental hospital, next to a building that housed chronically ill patients. He stored the urine samples he collected from patients in his family's refrigerator. He had no funding and no collaborators.

Nonetheless, this unassuming and seemingly ordinary man was, in certain ways, not ordinary at all. Cade was able to make his dis-covery not in spite of what was by today's standards a meager and seemingly unsupportive scientific environment but because of it.

Cade's discovery of lithium's therapeutic value was not, as some have suggested, a matter of luck; rather, it rested on an exceptional combination of Cade's life experiences, his personal and intellec-tual qualities, and the environment in which he worked.

Cade's keen awareness of the necessity for effective psychiatric treatment was forged early. His physician father worked as the medical superintendent of several mental hospitals. As a result, the Cade family lived on the grounds of these hospitals, and John

Cade and his two brothers grew up among mental patients. The years spent among these patients left Cade with a singular empathy for them.

Like his father, Cade trained to be a physician, and like his father, he went to war soon after completing his medical training, enlisting in the Australian Army in World War II. Captured on the island of Singapore in February 1942, Cade spent three and a half years as a Japanese prisoner of war on the island, at the notorious Changi Prison. Although Cade's official position in the army was general medical officer, because of his psychiatric training he was put in charge of Changi's psychiatric ward. In that capacity he observed and attempted to treat a wide range of mental problems with the limited resources he had at hand. Cade became convinced that at least some of these problems were a result of malnutrition. Cade's belief that mental ills have their roots in bodily changes was reinforced by the brain abnormalities he saw when he carried out autopsies on prisoners who had suffered mental disturbances.

The years he spent in Changi fueled Cade's desire to find an effective treatment for mental illness. Having nothing of substance to offer the many POWs who suffered depression, Cade became painfully aware of his field's lack of therapeutic tools. He subsequently devoted his career to caring for, and seeking treatments for, the chronically and severely mentally ill. "I returned from three and a half years as a prisoner of war," Cade said, "mourning the wasted years and determined to pursue the ideas that had germinated in that interminable time."[2]

Cade's childhood experiences, curiosity, courage, intelligence, perseverance, and powers of observation all figured in his lithium discovery. But the postwar environment in which he worked also played a part. Unencumbered by the necessity to write grant proposals or to publish lest he perish, he was able to pursue a research idea for an extended period of time and follow the clues that his observations provided. Unencumbered, as well, by the demands of third-party payers to limit the length of patient hospital stays, he had the time to properly implement his new treatment and observe its effects.

Thirty years after his lithium discovery Cade remarked, "I was able to go my own way unhindered by advice, criticism or caution. This is important. I don't think it could happen these days. One would be suffocated by hospital boards, research committees, ethical committees and heads of departments. Instead I was answerable only to my own conscience and personal drive."[3]

Cade is acknowledged as the originator of lithium treatment. It is likely, in fact, that without him lithium's value as a treatment for manic-depressive illness would never have been discovered. After all, there is no scientific reason to suspect that this simple element would alleviate the symptoms of mania. Even now, though scientists understand far more about how lithium works on brain cells than they did in Cade's day, they still cannot explain how it curbs mania. And although, in the century before Cade's discovery, lithium had been used for a number of medical and psychiatric ills—including gout, depression, and epilepsy—and mineral baths containing high concentrations of lithium had been thought to have general curative powers, by the time Cade came along, lithium had been abandoned as a treatment for anything.

But this is not a straightforward story of discovery and one inspired scientist. Not long after his 1949 landmark paper on lithium appeared and psychiatrists in Australia had started to use the drug, Cade himself declared that lithium was dangerous and should not be prescribed; one of his first patients treated with lithium had subsequently died, and two other deaths in lithium-treated patients were reported. In 1952, concerned that lithium was too toxic for clinical use, Cade, now superintendent of Melbourne's prestigious Royal Park Mental Hospital, prohibited its use there.

Cade's dire warnings, along with the widely publicized deaths and not infrequent toxic reactions to lithium might well have spelled the end of the drug. But other scientists came to the rescue. Edward Trautner, a refugee from Nazi Germany who was in the department of physiology and pharmacology at the University of Melbourne, was one. He realized that he could measure blood levels of lithium using flame photometry. A colleague in a nearby laboratory had set up this technique just the year before in order to measure the constituents of blood in sheep. Trautner and one of his former students launched a large study of lithium-treated patients, published in 1951, in which they measured lithium levels and carefully monitored and adjusted the lithium dose. They confirmed Cade's observation that lithium alleviated mania, and they showed as well that it could be given safely; none of the 100 patients in their study suffered serious intoxication and none died. In this and subsequent studies, Trautner and his colleagues identified a specific lithium blood-level range necessary for both safety and effectiveness. Today, patients taking lithium undergo regular blood tests to ensure that their lithium levels are in the range identified by Trautner and his colleagues.

Although Trautner's work made it possible for lithium to be widely studied and prescribed, his contributions have barely been acknowledged. Cade, in discussing the development of lithium decades after its importance was recognized and he was acclaimed as its discoverer, failed to mention Trautner's contribution. Whether this was a simple oversight or a deliberate attempt on Cade's part to take an inordinate share of the credit remains unclear, and in the psychopharmacology community, it is still a matter of controversy.

A Danish psychiatrist named Mogens Schou was the other major figure in the lithium story. In 1953, having recently joined the staff of Denmark's Aarhus University Psychiatric Hospital as a research associate, Schou was looking for a project. His chief, intrigued by Cade's and Trautner's lithium work, suggested that Schou investigate the claim that lithium alleviates the symptoms of mania. At that point, although the lithium studies from Australia certainly seemed to show that lithium curtails mania, they did not provide definitive proof; such proof, and lithium's acceptance as a treatment, required "controlled" research in which lithium was compared with no treatment, a placebo, or a different treatment. Schou set about to do just that sort of research. In a series of methodical studies, Schou and his collaborators confirmed that lithium is in fact an effective treatment for mania. More importantly, Schou and his collaborators showed that lithium can prevent episodes of both mania and depression. This prophylactic effect of lithium is recognized today as its most important benefit, and Cade readily acknowledged Schou's contributions.

Schou's work provided the basis for lithium's acceptance as a treatment. It was widely confirmed by other researchers and has been validated by more than five decades of clinical experience. Yet Schou—and lithium—did not have an easy time of it. Schou's early studies were criticized—attacked might be more accurate—by psychiatrists at London's prestigious Maudsley Hospital. Decades before "evidence-based medicine" became the watchword of the day, the Maudsley prided itself on rigorous evaluation of alleged treatments. And, in fact, Maudsley psychiatrists had debunked a number of bogus treatments. But they weren't always right.

Two Maudsley psychiatrists claimed that the idea, based on Schou's studies, that lithium has a prophylactic effect was a "myth." They reproached Schou for not using sufficiently rigorous control methodology. Some of the methodological fine points they raised were legitimate matters for debate. But the criticism took on an ad hominem tone. The Maudsley psychiatrists claimed that Schou was biased in favor of lithium's preventive benefit because he had treated his brother, who had suffered intractable recurrent depression, with lithium and was convinced that lithium had cured him, transforming his life. The ensuing storm, known among psychopharmacology insiders as the "Battle of Britain" was resolved over the ensuing decade only after further studies by Schou and others confirmed the initial findings.

The place of lithium in the treatment of bipolar disorder is now well established and the contributions of Cade and others to its discovery and development generally acknowledged. Over the past few decades, a few other drugs appeared to be supplanting lithium or at least challenging its predominance, largely because they were heavily promoted by the pharmaceutical industry. Not patentable and inexpensive, lithium has never been marketed and no single company is motivated to promote it. But lithium's advantages over its patented, profitable, and well-advertised competitors are becoming more apparent. In addition to the fact that lithium may simply be more effective than other so-called mood stabilizers in preventing episodes of illness in bipolar patients, lithium offers the unique benefit of drastically reducing suicide in these patients. Lithium also continues to be tested in other conditions characterized by extreme fluctuations in mood and behavior. What's more, lithium's specificity and effectiveness for manic depression render it an important research tool in the quest to uncover the causes of the illness.

Lithium treatment has been available for about 60 years, but manic-depressive illness has been with us since antiquity. We begin our story with this illness and the plight of those afflicted with it before lithium came on the scene.

LITHIUM

---|---

Manic-Depressive Illness,
A Brief History

IN 1378, Pope Gregory XI—the seventh and last of the popes to reign from the French city of Avignon—died. Nine days after his death, when the red-cloaked cardinals swept into the Vatican to elect a new pontiff, they were faced with a fuming crowd demanding that the next pope be Roman or, at the very least, Italian. Members of the mob stole into the palace and tried to extort a promise to that effect. The next morning, the assembled cardinals hurriedly conceded to the pressure; they selected Bartolomeo Prignano, the Archbishop of Bari. Prignano had been a monk and then a respected administrator in the papal chancery at Avignon. At the time of his election, his contemporaries described him as "learned, modest and devout."[1] He took the name of Urban VI. Soon after his coronation, however, Urban VI showed a drastic change in behavior. He became volatile, angry, and abusive, berating the cardinals both individually and collectively and getting into brawls with those who visited to pay homage. He made extravagant statements, among them that he could now depose kings and emperors. Summing up Urban's faults, the church historian Ludwig von Pastor wrote, "He lacked Christian gentleness and charity. He was naturally arbitrary and extremely violent and imprudent."[2]

Not surprisingly, the cardinals had second thoughts about their newly chosen leader. They asked Urban VI to resign and held a second election. Also not surprisingly, Urban VI flatly refused to step down. For the next 40 years, there were two rival lines of popes, elected by the same College of Cardinals. The Great Schism of 1378–1418, with its attendant conflicts and corruption, diminished the prestige and power of the papacy.

Although tagging a figure from the past with a psychiatric diagnosis is an iffy business, Urban VI's behavior is certainly characteristic of the manic phase of manic-depressive illness. No less an authority than John Cade suggested that manic-depressive mood swings in key leaders have altered the course of history. He proposed that in the case of Urban VI, later known to history as the "Mad Pope," manic-depressive illness contributed to the Protestant Reformation.[3]

Whether or not manic-depressive illness was responsible for shaking the primacy of the Catholic Church and the historical paroxysms that followed, there is no doubt that it has been with us since antiquity, that it has affected millions of people (about 1 percent of the population), that it strikes all nations, cultures, and social classes, and that it is among the most devastating afflictions. In addition to Urban VI, we now suspect that a good number of other famous figures suffered from this illness, including Robert Schumann, Abraham Lincoln, Winston Churchill, and Ernest Hemingway.[4]

What we know as manic-depressive illness or bipolar disorder was described in the writings of Hippocrates and his school in about 400 BCE. The ancient Greeks applied the term *melancholia* to the crushing despondency, lethargy, and hopelessness that we now call severe depression. According to Hippocrates's humoral system of medicine, health and disease depended on the proper balance of four body fluids, or humors: blood, phlegm, yellow bile, and black bile. Melancholia (from *melos*, meaning black, and *choler*, meaning bile) was thought to result from an excess of black bile.

The term *mania* also comes from the ancient Greeks. Unlike the term *melancholia*, which described pretty much the same thing in ancient Greece as it does today, in ancient times the term *mania* described a variety of conditions marked by excitement and irrational behavior. One of them was the state of exuberance, extreme activity, euphoria, and rage that we now call mania. But the term *mania* or *maniac* was also applied to the delirium of intoxication and the excitement and agitation associated with fever and brain diseases. Within the humoral theory, mania arose from an excess of yellow bile or a mixture of black and yellow bile.

Despite a total lack of evidence to support it, the humoral theory dominated medical thinking for more than 2,000 years. It was not fully displaced until the mid-nineteenth century, when scientifically based pathology came on the scene. Yet before we get too self-congratulatory about how far we've come from the ancients in our knowledge of disease, it's worth noting that there are still remnants of the humoral theory in contemporary medicine. Doctors refer to humoral immunity when describing antibodies that help fight disease and circulate in body fluids. And the idea of balance, a key feature of the humoral theory, is still part of our modern concept of a healthy lifestyle.

People who suffered bouts of both melancholia and mania have been described in medical writings since antiquity, and although these conditions were generally considered separate afflictions, a number of medical writers from ancient times alluded to a link between them. In the first century CE, the Greek physician Aretaeus of Cappadocia described a group of patients who "laugh, play, dance night and day, and sometimes go openly to the market crowned, as if victors in some contest of skill," only to be "torpid, dull, and sorrowful" at other times.[5] In his book on medical psychology, *Two Discourses Concerning the Soul of Brutes*, originally published in Latin in 1672, Thomas Willis, the celebrated neuroanatomist and physician, wrote: "Manics and melancholics are so much akin, that these Distempers often change, and pass from one into the other, for the Melancholick disposition growing worse, brings on Fury; and Fury or Madness growing less hot, oftentimes ends in a Melancholick disposition."[6] It was not until the mid-nineteenth century, however, that mania and melancholia were clearly and explicitly recognized as different phases of one illness.

On January 31, 1854, in the vaulted hall of the Hospital of Charity on Rue Saint Pierre in Paris, the French psychiatrist Jules Baillarger gave a lecture to the French Imperial Academy of Medicine in which he described a mental illness characterized by recurrent oscillations between mania and depression. He named this illness *folie a double forme* (dual-form insanity). Two weeks later, on February 14, 1854, Jean-Pierre Falret, another French psychiatrist, presented a description to the academy of what was essentially the same illness. He named it *folie circulaire* (circular insanity). The two went on to bitterly dispute who had been the first to conceptualize the disorder. Falret claimed that he had been describing *folie circulaire* for years in his lectures at the Salpêtrière, the renowned Paris asylum. Whoever came first, both men described the essential features of what came to be known as manic-depressive illness and, later, bipolar disorder. They pointed out that the illness has two phases, mania and depression, that the phases can follow each other in rapid succession or be separated by years, and that the phases recur with varying degrees of frequency, depending on the patient. Although historians of psychiatry now credit Baillarger and Falret with being the first to come up with the modern concept of what became known as manic-depressive illness, their presentations and later publications on the matter had little impact at the time. Their terms for the disorder were never widely used, and their work did not appear to influence the nineteenth- and early twentieth-century psychiatrists who further described the symptoms and course of the same illness.

It was the renowned German psychiatrist and nosologist Emil Kraepelin (1856–1926) who put manic-depressive illness on the map and established it as one of the major mental disorders. Widely regarded as the founder of modern psychiatry, Kraepelin developed a method for classifying psychiatric disorders, still in use today, which is based on the pattern of symptoms and the course of the disorder over time. Among his other contributions, he recognized that hundreds of psychiatric disorders then categorized as separate illnesses were in fact a single disease entity, which he termed *dementia praecox*, now called schizophrenia. In 1899, in the sixth edition of his legendary psychiatric textbook, he coined the term *manic-depressive insanity* and provided a description of its symptoms and course, a description that remains the basis of its diagnosis to this day. Kraepelin emphasized the recurrent nature of this illness and noted that between periods of mania and depression, patients were free of symptoms and able to function normally.

Kraepelin's landmark conceptualization of manic-depressive illness continues to dominate psychiatric thinking, but since Kraepelin's day, we've discovered several varieties of this illness and filled in details of its symptoms and course. On average, a person with untreated manic-depressive illness has an episode of mania or depression about every two years. A sizable minority experience what is called rapid cycling, four or more manic or depressive episodes per year, and a few people switch from mania to depression and back within just one or two days. In the 1970s, psychiatric researchers found that some people have recurrent depressions and also have occasional periods of high energy, ebullience, and increased activity—but of lesser severity than mania and technically known as hypomania. This condition has been termed bipolar II disorder (the archetypal manic-depressive illness described by Baillarger, Falret, and Kraepelin is designated bipolar I).

Although the symptoms of manic-depressive illness are the same now as they were in antiquity, the terms we use to describe this disorder have varied over the years and reflect contemporary fashions in psychiatric diagnosis and concepts of disease causation. For example, while the term *depression* had occasionally been used as far back as the eighteenth century to describe a state of lassitude and demoralization, *melancholia* was the customary designation from ancient times until the early twentieth century. In the fifth edition of his psychiatric textbook (1896), Kraepelin abandoned *melancholia* for *depression*, and in 1904, Adolph Meyer, the dean of American psychiatry, explicitly recommended that the term *melancholia* be eliminated from the psychiatric lexicon and replaced with *depression*. He objected to *melancholia* because it implied that we had knowledge of the cause of the illness, which, in fact, we did not. Black bile is not, after all, the root of the affliction.

With the prestige of Kraepelin and Meyer behind this change, the worldwide psychiatric community discarded *melancholia* in favor of *depression*. I, and a good number of my colleagues, believe that this was a mistake. *Depression* is such a nonspecific term that when a patient of mine tells me that he was depressed last year, it's unclear if he was sad for a day or two or if he had the unrelenting lethargy and despair that comes with the depressive phase of bipolar disorder.

As William Styron wrote in *Darkness Visible*, his memoir about his struggle with depression, "'Melancholia' would still appear to be a far more apt and evocative word for the blacker forms of the disorder, but it was usurped by a noun with a bland tonality and lacking any magisterial presence, used indifferently to describe an economic decline or a rut in the ground, a true wimp of a word for such a major illness."[7]

Manic-depressive illness became officially known as bipolar disorder in 1980 with the introduction of the third edition of the American Psychiatric Association's diagnostic and statistical manual (DSM III). In Kraepelin's original conceptualization, manic-depressive illness included any periodic disorder of mood, including recurrent episodes of just depression as well as episodes of both depression and mania. The committee that updated the diagnostic manual believed that recurrent depressions and recurrent episodes of both mania and depression were different "diseases" and came up with the terms *unipolar depression* and *bipolar disorder* to differentiate them. In addition, the committee felt that *bipolar disorder* was a less stigmatizing term than *manic-depressive illness* because it avoided the word *manic* with its similarity to *maniac*. Although *bipolar disorder* has been the conventional diagnostic term for almost 40 years, the matter of whether recurrent depressions and recurrent episodes of both mania and depression are different diseases or variants of the same disease remains unsettled. There are experts on both sides of this debate. Genetic and treatment studies lean toward the one-disease notion; and we cannot easily dismiss the fact that Kraepelin considered them one disease. After all, he was right about all sorts of stuff, including his now widely accepted idea that the course of an illness and its outcome are more telling indicators of a psychiatric disease than are individual symptoms.

Despite great advances in our understanding of the brain, and despite thousands of studies examining the brains of people with manic-depressive illness, we know little more about the causes of manic-depressive illness now than we did in the time of Hippocrates. The humoral theory continues to dominate our notions of what causes depression and mania, albeit in a present-day disguise. For example, depression and mania are widely believed by both medical professionals and the general public to result from a deficiency or excess of brain neurotransmitters, the chemicals that carry signals from one nerve cell to another. The idea that too little or too much of one of these brain chemicals causes depression or mania appeared about 50 years ago, is based on scanty evidence, is at best a vast oversimplification, and is probably incorrect. Experts in brain chemistry no longer endorse this notion. But it has intuitive appeal—too little brain juice gets you depressed, too much and you're manic—and has dominated our concepts of what causes manic-depressive illness for the last half-century.

The widely touted serotonin theory of depression, that too little of this neurotransmitter causes depression, does not rest on an appreciably firmer scientific base than the black bile and yellow bile business. The only rationale for the theory is that drugs that affect serotonin can alleviate depression. But the antidepressants that increase serotonin also do many other things in the brain—including stimulating nerve growth—any one of which might be the reason they ease depression. What's more, some drugs that are effective antidepressants don't influence serotonin levels. If a serotonin deficiency truly were responsible for depression, these drugs would not work.

Although we are still far from pinpointing the basis of manic-depressive illness, today we do have some persuasive clues. The first big clue comes from the families of people with the illness.

The fact that the close relatives of people with manic-depressive illness are 10 times more likely than the general population to have this condition has been known for more than 100 years. But until the latter half of the twentieth century and the advent of sophisticated family and genetic studies, it wasn't clear whether the high prevalence of the illness in some families is a result of the family environment or whether it results from the sharing of a certain genetic constitution. It is now clear that shared genes account for the high prevalence of manic-depressive illness within certain families, whereas environmental factors, such as location, diet, and style of parental upbringing, play a negligible role, if any.

How do we know? Although several types of family studies pointed to the importance of genetic constitution, or the primacy of "nature" over "nurture," the studies that proved the essential role of genes were comparisons of concordance rates in identical and fraternal twins. Disease concordance means the likelihood that one twin has the same condition as the other. Because identical twins, technically known as monozygotic twins, come from the same fertilized egg, or zygote, they have similar genes. Fraternal, or dizygotic, twins come from two different eggs and are genetically different. So if the concordance rate for a certain illness is higher in identical than in fraternal twins, then the illness in question has a clear genetic component. Studies that have compared concordance rates for manic-depressive illness in identical and fraternal twins have found that if one identical twin has manic-depressive illness, the other one also has it about 60 percent of the time; the concordance rate for fraternal twins is far lower, at about 10 percent.[8]

Twin concordance studies are an elegant way to separate the influences of environment and genes. Because identical and fraternal twins share the same family environment, a difference in the concordance rates for manic-depressive illness between the two types of twins means that genetics is clearly at play. Unfortunately, our knowledge doesn't go much further.

Researchers have been trying to identify the specific genes that increase risk for manic-depressive illness for more than 30 years, but so far these genes have been elusive. It does seem clear that unlike the case for some diseases that are clearly genetically based, such as cystic fibrosis, Huntington disease, and Down syndrome, manic-depressive illness does not arise from a major aberration in one gene or chromosome (a cellular structure that contains specific genes). Rather, it seems likely that smaller anomalies in several genes combine to create risk for the illness. Almost every year genetic studies of manic-depressive illness identify several genes that seem to be associated with the illness in one or more families, only to find that with further analysis or additional studies the association fails to hold up.

The Old Order Amish study is a case in point.[9] As a graduate student in the 1960s, Janice Egeland was studying health behaviors and beliefs within Old Order Amish communities in central Pennsylvania. In the course of her work, she learned that several large families had multiple members with manic-depressive illness. The Amish community was very aware of this condition and in fact was convinced that it was heritable. They called it "siss im blut," German for "in the blood." In 1976, Egeland, then a professor of psychiatry and epidemiology, launched an epidemiological and genetic study of manic-depressive illness among the Old Order Amish. That study continued for more than 30 years. Although the Amish do not participate fully in our high-tech world, they were nevertheless eager to take part in this study; it had the potential to advance knowledge of a condition that obviously troubled many in their community and about which they had unanswered questions.

The Amish are ideal subjects for genetic studies. They are descended from about 30 pioneer couples who came to the United States from Switzerland in the 1700s. There is little migration into the community—few people convert to the Amish way of life. They are what is known as a genetic isolate, and accordingly, they display much less genetic variability than the general population. Amish also tend to have large families, and they keep extensive genealogical records. All these factors facilitate the identification of genetic markers that may be related to an illness.

Any genetic study of bipolar disorder stands or falls on the accuracy with which people afflicted with the disorder are identified. The Old Order Amish are ideal subjects in this regard as well; they prohibit alcohol and other drugs, the use of which can obscure the diagnosis of bipolar disorder in the general population, and their strict standards of behavior make the unusual behavior of a manic or depressive episode easy to recognize. Whereas typical features of a manic episode in the general population—excessive shopping, middle-of-the-night housecleaning, nonstop bar hopping and sexual promiscuity—can often be difficult to differentiate from normal behavior, the typical features of such an episode in an Amish community—driving a horse and buggy too fast, using electrical machinery or buying a car—are easily recognized in the community as aberrant.

Egeland and her team conducted detailed psychiatric interviews of the members of five large multigenerational families in which there was a pattern of bipolar disorder over several generations. They also took blood samples for DNA analysis from family members with and without the illness. In 1987, they found in one of these families a DNA marker that was associated with manic-depressive illness. The results, reported in *Nature*, the leading scientific journal, electrified the scientific community.[10] It seemed that Egeland's team had revealed for the first time the genetic foundation of a psychiatric illness. Egeland and her discovery received worldwide acclaim. She was showered with prizes and accolades. An international psychiatric genetics conference honored Egeland as one of three scientists who achieved the biggest breakthroughs of the twentieth century.

Enthralled by the implications of Egeland's discovery, I invited her to give a lecture at Brown University, where I was on the faculty, immersed in my own research on the biological basis of psychiatric disorders. I introduced Egeland as someone who for the first time in history had uncovered the biological basis of a mental disorder—manic-depressive illness—and set psychiatry on a new footing.

Her triumph, however, was short-lived. Until a finding is replicated, it is not considered solid, and upon further analysis of the same Amish family over the next two years, Egeland and her team were unable to replicate their initial findings. When they included several new family members, the link between the DNA marker and manic-depressive illness was no longer sufficiently powerful to meet statistical standards. In 1989, they reported these negative— and disappointing—results in *Nature*.[11]

Although the Amish gene for manic-depressive illness proved elusive, as have many other candidate genes since, the Amish study was not a wasted effort. It provided information about the prevalence of manic-depressive illness and about early signs of this illness in children. Amish children's lives are so structured and their household responsibilities so well defined that any deviation is instantly noticeable. The study also highlighted some of the problems encountered in conducting this sort of family research, such as accurately identifying affected family members, and the importance of applying rigorous methods of diagnosis and statistical analysis. The methodological refinements that came out of the Amish study have informed the current generation of genetics studies.

Despite astounding advances in DNA technology and the hope that these advances would soon lead to solid information on the genetics of manic-depressive illness, this goal is far from being realized. And it's worth noting that the identification of one or more gene abnormalities in people with bipolar disorder is just the first step in uncovering the basis of this disorder. Aberrant or faulty genes produce diseases by making abnormal proteins that then interfere with the functioning of certain cells, organs, and other body tissues. So even if unmistakable gene abnormalities were identified in people with bipolar disorder, the tasks of discovering the atypical proteins these genes produce and then the way these proteins affect the functioning of the body would remain. There is, in short, a lot of work to be done.

The second big clue about the basis of manic-depressive illness comes from the fact that its symptoms can be alleviated and, most importantly, *prevented* by lithium. Lithium is a naturally occurring element, a light metal found throughout earth in the form of one of its salts. Although there are plenty of drugs that can lighten the apathy of depression and quiet the excesses of mania, lithium does so without producing sedation or other psychological side effects, and it is unique in its ability to prevent these episodes. People with manic-depressive illness who respond to lithium, and most do, lead essentially normal lives, free of devastating mood swings. If we understood how lithium prevents these episodes, we would be well on our way to understanding what causes them. We know that lithium has an impact on numerous bodily processes, including the activity of enzymes, molecules necessary for our cells to operate properly. We know a good deal about what these processes are and how lithium alters them. What we don't know is which of lithium's many cellular effects accounts for its powerful healing properties.

Prior to 1949, when John Cade made his breakthrough discovery that lithium alleviates the symptoms of mania, there was no effective treatment for manic-depressive illness. Electroconvulsive therapy (ECT), discovered in 1938, was and still remains a good treatment for melancholia, and it could quiet a frenzied manic patient. But the results were often temporary. Further, ECT, which entailed the electrical induction of seizures, had troublesome side effects in Cade's day. When we give ECT today, we also provide medications that eliminate actual convulsions; in Cade's day, however, patients undergoing ECT had severe spasms and contractions that often resulted in broken bones and other injuries. Some patients also experienced memory loss, as they sometimes do today.

The absence of effective treatments for manic-depressive illness in earlier times did not mean that these patients were not treated. They were treated with all sorts of substances and procedures from ancient times onward. It's just that none of these treatments worked, and most were harmful.

Some of the earliest treatments, in place well before the Middle Ages, were applied to people with any type of mental or behavioral disturbance, including melancholia and mania. Physicians of old made liberal use of bleeding and purging in people with mental disorders. Like all treatments, whether truly effective or not, these came with a compelling rationale. Bleeding was thought to remove toxins and restore the balance of humors. It was the longest-lasting treatment in medicine, used for more than 2,000 years and not abandoned until the early twentieth century.

Insanity was thought to result from toxins residing in the colon; hence, purging with laxatives was an integral part of psychiatric treatment. Through the 1920s, in fact, English psychiatrists continued to rely on croton oil, a powerful purgative, "to abort or cut short a mental crisis."[12] Laxatives as a treatment for mental illness fell out of favor by the middle of the twentieth century as it became clear that the colonic toxin theory was wrong and as truly effective treatments for mental disorders came to the fore. Nonetheless, although there is no scientific evidence that laxatives or other forms of purging provide health benefits, colonic cleansing remains a staple of today's alternative medicine; its adherents claim that it benefits a wide range of ailments from arthritis to anxiety. And like the ancient Egyptians and Greeks, who developed the toxins-in-the-colon theory of disease, many today continue to believe that the intestines harbor all sorts of mischief; one does not have to go far beyond friends and family to find people who think that daily bowel evacuation is necessary for health and that constipation brings all sorts of trouble.

Opium was one of the few ancient treatments that actually had some inherent therapeutic value. It was used from ancient times as a sedative and pain reliever, and it worked. The Ebers Papyrus from 1500 BCE provides details on how to "stop a crying child" using the grains of a poppy plant.[13] Until modern times, opium was also used as a cure-all; in the seventeenth century, Thomas Sydenham, the renowned English physician, reflected the prevailing medical opinion when he wrote, "Among the remedies which it has pleased Almighty God to give to man to relieve his sufferings, none is so universal and so efficacious as opium."[14]

Although opium did sedate and calm agitated and anxious people, it had little effect on major mental illnesses like schizophrenia and manic-depressive illness. Nevertheless, until the mid-twentieth century and the discovery of effective psychiatric drugs, opium, and later other sedatives, were the only drugs on hand. So that's what manic-depressive patients got—opium and its derivatives, bromides and barbiturates. In dangerously high doses, these sedatives could put both melancholic and manic patients to sleep, but otherwise they did nothing to alleviate the symptoms of this illness.

Until the Middle Ages, families were responsible for the management of the mentally ill. If mentally ill people were not disruptive, they were left to their own devices, free to wander about or talk quietly to themselves. It is estimated that about 20 percent of people with untreated manic-depressive illness commit suicide, so it's probably safe to assume that before the modern era, a substantial portion of manic-depressive patients killed themselves. Although the depressive phase of manic-depressive illness left people unable to care for themselves or contribute to family life, it was the manic phase with its frenzied activity, irrational talk, and bizarre conduct that prompted families to apply extreme means of restraint. People with these sorts of disorderly symptoms were confined in cages, chained to walls, or locked in tiny rooms, stables, and stalls.

In 1817, a member of the British House of Commons from an Irish district described the plight of a mentally ill person in the cabin of an Irish peasant family. When a family member develops madness, he said, "the only way they have to manage is by making a hole in the floor of the cabin, not high enough for the person to stand up in, with a crib over it to prevent his getting up. This hole is about five feet deep, and they give this wretched being his food there, and there he generally dies."[15]

Although asylums started to appear in the Middle Ages, families continued to provide much of the custodial care for people with mental afflictions, including manic-depressive illness, until well into the nineteenth century. The early asylums were confined to cities and housed a diverse population of the unwanted, including vagrants, criminals, the mentally retarded, and the mentally ill. These early asylums were essentially prisons; they did not pretend to offer any sort of treatment. Inmates were frequently chained and beaten; various forms of restraint, including straitjackets and confinement in cages and small rooms, were the order of the day.

Starting in the late eighteenth century, in the midst of the French Revolution and in concert with its ideals, asylums underwent a major transformation. The value that the Enlightenment placed on innovation and the humanitarian principles of the revolution set the stage for and prompted major reforms at the Bicêtre and Salpêtrière, the renowned Paris asylums, and these reforms spread throughout Europe and the United States. Patients were unchained, and the use of physical restraints and padded cells was limited. The directors and staffs of the asylums began to look upon people with mental illness as warranting treatment, not simply incarceration. This shift in attitude evolved into "moral treatment"; asylums became healing environments that provided pleasant surroundings, good food, soothing conversation, and opportunities for work and quiet activities. According to the records of the time, patients often improved in this environment and were able to return to their families.

Along with beautiful gardens and walking paths, the asylums and retreats of the nineteenth century incorporated a number of procedures designed to calm and control agitated and excited patients. These included hot and cold baths and cold wet sheet packs. The wet sheet pack, in which an agitated patient is tightly wrapped in a cold wet sheet or blanket, was applied well into the mid-twentieth century, and barbaric as it sounds, it is an extraordinarily effective calming method. As a last resort, the asylums of the nineteenth century used straitjackets and confined patients in padded cells.

Moral treatment fell into decline by the twentieth century. Although it was certainly a more benevolent approach than that of the early asylums, it didn't actually work all that well. Despite its intuitive appeal and the good intentions of its advocates, recovery rates were not as high as the early statistics suggested. Many people with serious mental disorders, including manic-depressive illness, had to be readmitted soon after discharge. Further, by the late nineteenth century, the asylums were overcrowded, and the activities and attentiveness integral to moral treatment were difficult to implement.

Moral treatment rested on the belief that people with mental disorders were curable and that gentle reeducation to alter their thinking and attitudes could restore them to health. By the end of the nineteenth century, these ideas had given way to the view that mental disorders were hereditary, that they involved malfunction of the brain or other organs, and that they were often enduring.

By the beginning of the twentieth century, with the demise of moral treatment and the great increase in the population of asylums, particularly public ones, these institutions had largely reverted to their pre-nineteenth-century custodial role with an emphasis on security, closed doors, and physical restraint. But the asylums of the early twentieth century differed in an important way from their predecessors: they introduced an astonishing variety of physical "treatments." Most did more harm than good, but they established psychiatry as a medical endeavor and supported the notion that serious mental illness had a biological basis.

The first of these treatments was malarial (fever) therapy for general paralysis of the insane (GPI), a brutal disorder of the brain caused by late-stage syphilis and involving relentless destruction of brain tissue. People with this condition made up a large share of asylum residents. A consequence of untreated syphilis, this infection of the brain resulted in, along with muscle paralysis, a wide array of mental symptoms, including hallucinations, delusions, depression, personality changes, and dementia.

Julius Wagner-Jauregg, a Viennese psychiatrist, had noticed that patients suffering with GPI sometimes improved after having a fever. He concluded that since the improvement occurred irrespective of the type of illness causing the fever, it was the high fever itself that brought about the recovery. Consistent with this observation, laboratory research had shown that the bug (*Treponema pallidum*) that causes syphilis is extraordinarily sensitive to heat; a few degrees above normal body temperature kills it. Wagner-Jauregg tested various methods of inducing fever in GPI patients without much success until, in 1917, he tried inducing malaria by injecting the blood of malarial patients. Of the first nine patients in whom Wagner-Jauregg produced malarial attacks (typically associated with high fevers), six showed substantial improvement and three were still alive and well 10 years later; without this treatment, all nine would have been long dead.[16] Malarial treatment became the standard treatment for GPI until penicillin came along in the mid-1940s. The discovery that malarial therapy was notably effective in treating this heretofore incurable disease reinforced the idea that mental symptoms could be cured by a physical treatment. For his discovery of malarial treatment, Wagner-Jauregg won the Nobel Prize in 1927.

Prolonged deep sleep was a popular treatment for a few years in the 1920s. Agitated patients with psychotic symptoms, including those with mania, were given high doses of barbiturates to induce deep sleep lasting about five days. When the patients awoke, they were often calm and rational. But the improvement usually didn't last, and a substantial number of patients died from pneumonia and other medical complications.

The 1920s also saw the rise and fall of one of the most gruesome treatments in the history of psychiatry. In the wake of the triumph of bacterial concepts of disease in the late nineteenth century, some clinicians theorized that mental illnesses, like schizophrenia and manic-depressive illness, might have an infectious origin. Prominent physicians in Europe and the United States embraced the idea that insanity resulted from toxins produced by untreated infections. Adolph Meyer, the foremost American psychiatrist and head of psychiatry at Johns Hopkins, was a strong advocate of this view. For the most part, this idea remained just that: an idea, prompting discussion and speculation.

But Doctor Henry Cotton, the superintendent of New Jersey State Hospital in Trenton from 1907 to 1930, put this notion into practice. And he did so with a vengeance bordering on the demonic. On the grounds that teeth harbored hidden infections, he and his staff began extracting the teeth of the mentally ill patients admitted to the hospital. When teeth extractions failed to elicit cures, Cotton went on to remove the patients' tonsils and thereafter began removing other organs that presumably might harbor infections, including stomachs, intestines, testicles, ovaries, gallbladders, cervices and, most of all, colons. Thousands of patients underwent these surgical procedures regardless of their objections; patients with manic-depressive illness were among the prime targets.

Cotton claimed that 85 percent of the patients recovered as a result of the surgery. He received worldwide accolades for applying seemingly state-of-the-art scientific methods to the treatment of mental illness. Patients and their families clamored to be treated at Trenton State. In 1922, the *New York Times* wrote: "At the State Hospital at Trenton, N.J., under the brilliant leadership of the medical director, Dr Henry A Cotton, there is on foot the most searching, aggressive, and profound scientific investigation that has yet been made of the whole field of nervous and mental disorders . . . there is hope, high hope . . . for the future."[17]

Despite the praise heaped on Cotton, not all psychiatrists believed that local infections were the cause of serious mental illness, and many questioned the benefits of surgery. A person could live without the organ that Cotton might deem infected and mark for removal, but before the discovery of antibiotics, surgery was inherently dangerous, and a high proportion of the patients subjected to Cotton's surgeries died. In his published papers, Cotton reported death rates of about 30 percent, but later scrutiny of his statistics revealed that the mortality rate was closer to 45 percent. Finally, a series of investigations in the mid-1920s cast doubt on all of Cotton's reported results. The statistics kept by Cotton and his staff turned out to be dodgy at best; "cure rates" were nowhere near 85 percent.

In retrospect, when a few patients did seem to improve after having their colons or testicles removed, it's clear that the surgery itself was not the reason. The symptoms of many mental disorders, most notably manic-depressive illness, wax and wane. Even without treatment, patients in the throes of mania or depression usually recuperate within three to six months. So when any treatment seems to provide a cure for manic-depressive illness, spontaneous recovery may be at play. A control group—patients who don't receive treatment and who are compared with those who do— can help tease out spontaneous recovery and placebo effect from the actual value of an experimental treatment. Although control groups are now an essential part of treatment research, they were not widely applied in Cotton's day.

The sorry tale of Cotton and his psychiatric surgery has a suitably tawdry ending. In the mid-1920s, Adolph Meyer commissioned Doctor Phyllis Greenacre, one of his former students, to conduct an independent analysis of Cotton's work. In her preliminary report, she expressed serious misgivings both about Cotton's methods and about his reported results. Meyer, who continued to believe, like Cotton, that hidden infections produce mental illness, suppressed Greenacre's report, preventing it from being completed or published.[18] Undeterred by Greenacre's damning findings and the equally damning findings of other investigations, Meyer continued to endorse Cotton's methods. Finally, with Cotton's retirement in 1930, the surgery at Trenton State came to an end. Happily, its lack of clear success and high mortality rates prevented it from ever being widely adopted. Greenacre went on to a distinguished career as a psychoanalyst.

Cotton and his surgical treatments are now thoroughly discredited. His therapeutic zeal was at best misguided, his insistence on the value of his surgeries bordered on the delusional, and, from today's perspective, subjecting patients to destructive surgery without their consent was unethical and cruel.

His tale is a cautionary one. Although hospital oversight committees of today do their best to protect the rights and welfare of patients, there is still plenty of room in the contemporary practice of medicine, including psychiatry, for risky and expensive treatments to be zealously applied in the absence of any reliable evidence for their value. As just one example, a number of new methods that deliver mild electric currents to the brain—such as vagus nerve stimulation, in which current is applied to the vagus nerve (a nerve that runs through the neck to the brain), and transcranial magnetic stimulation, in which current is applied to the scalp—are now used for the treatment of depression. These procedures are costly, have detrimental side effects, and, in the case of vagus nerve stimulation, require surgery; there is also no solid evidence for their effectiveness. Nevertheless, these treatments have enthusiastic advocates and are heavily promoted and widely applied.

Insulin coma therapy dominated psychiatric treatment in the 1930s. Similar in concept to deep sleep, patients were given increasing doses of insulin until their blood sugar fell dramatically and they entered a coma. After about 20 minutes in a coma, the patients got an infusion of glucose, which quickly restored them to consciousness. As was the case with deep sleep, when patients came out of the coma they were often free of troublesome symptoms, at least for a short time. Although asylum doctors used insulin coma therapy primarily for patients with schizophrenia, they also used it, with mixed results, in patients with manic-depressive illness, particularly those in the depressive phase.

Insulin coma therapy was difficult to implement and it was dangerous; if the coma went on for too long, the result could be brain damage or death. Comas were induced five times a week for weeks on end, and each required vigilance by hospital staff. Some patients did seem to benefit, but the results were hard to predict. With the arrival of electroconvulsive therapy (ECT) in the late 1930s, a procedure that was much easier to implement and produced equally good results, insulin coma therapy fell into decline. The death knell for insulin coma came with the discovery in the early 1950s of the phenothiazines—drugs that were clearly effective treatments for schizophrenia.

Electroconvulsive therapy is the only physical treatment developed in the first half of the twentieth century that has withstood the test of time and is still widely used. For reasons that remain baffling, when people with certain mental illnesses, notably schizophrenia and depression, undergo a seizure, they often get better. Ladislas von Meduna, a Hungarian psychiatrist, was the first to use seizures as a treatment. He had become convinced that people with schizophrenia improved after developing epilepsy and wondered if producing epileptic fits would therefore alleviate the symptoms of schizophrenia. In the early 1930s, he induced seizures with injections of the chemical metrazol and found that after several convulsions, patients with schizophrenia were often markedly better, free of irrational thinking and hallucinations. He and his colleagues went on to induce convulsions in people with other mental afflictions. Patients with melancholia also got better after a series of convulsions. Despite the extreme stress that convulsions placed on the heart and bones, not infrequently resulting in shoulder and jaw dislocations and fractures of the spine, convulsive treatment was widely embraced; it was plainly the best treatment yet for schizophrenia and depression. By 1935, convulsive therapy was extensively used in asylums. But the metrazol induction method was not ideal; it did not reliably produce seizures, and patients feared it. During the 30 or 40 seconds between the injection and the onset of convulsions, patients experienced intense anxiety to the point where they felt that death was imminent. And so, when in 1938 Ugo Cerletti, an Italian psychiatrist, discovered that an electric current applied to the head could more reliably and safely produce convulsions, that method quickly came to the fore. Electroconvulsive therapy remains an important treatment for manic-depressive illness when the currently available drugs don't work. It consistently brings people with melancholia out of their despair and, paradoxical as it sounds, can also quiet the patient in the throes of severe mania. Unfortunately, its benefits are temporary. Attacks of depression and mania invariably recur.

Lobotomy, also known as leucotomy, was the last of the physical treatments launched in the first half of the twentieth century, and from the beginning it was the most controversial. In a lobotomy, a surgeon severs the nerve fibers that connect the brain's frontal lobes to other parts of the brain. When normally connected, the frontal lobes supply a number of essential mental functions, including planning, motivation, memory, emotional expression, reasoning, and regulation of behavior. The idea that interfering with these connections could be a useful treatment for mental illness arose from the observation that people who undergo damage to their brain's frontal lobes often experience personality changes. Some of these changes are harmful: the victims of such injuries are typically less aware of the social niceties than before the injury and are sometimes intellectually impaired; but often they are more placid and agreeable as well.

In his 1979 book *Mending the Mind*, John Cade offered an example from World War I that foretold lobotomy's use as a treatment: "A melancholic major decided to end it all and put a neat through-and-through bullet hole through the frontal lobes of his brain with his service revolver. He was promptly evacuated to the regimental aid post, where the doctor was struck by and remembered for many years the patient's amazing composure, indeed contentment and complacence. He had blown his melancholia clean out of his head."[19]

These sorts of observations about frontal lobe injury—many of which involved wounds received in combat—along with the results of brain research in animals inspired Portuguese neurologist António Egas Moniz to undertake lobotomy as a treatment for mental illness. Moniz may have been particularly encouraged by a 1935 presentation at the Second International Neurological Congress, where he heard about two chimpanzees who had their frontal lobes removed and afterward were remarkably pacified. Three months later, Moniz started doing lobotomies on psychiatric patients. We don't know precisely what he and the surgeons who followed him told these patients or their families, but it's clear that the informed consent that is now such an important part of any treatment, particularly a new one, was not brought into play; patients more often than not had no say in the matter whatsoever.

Observations on the effects of frontal lobe damage did not seem to provide sufficient grounds for the application of lobotomy, so, like all treatments, lobotomy acquired a "scientific" rationale. The idea, cooked up by Moniz and others, was that certain forms of psychological distress, particularly severe obsessions and compulsions and unrelenting depression, resulted from neural pathways caught in fixed destructive circuits. Interrupting those pathways would relieve these unremitting symptoms. This belief rested on no actual knowledge of what was going on in the brain, but it provided Moniz and others with a scientific justification for subjecting mental patients to brain surgery.

Patients with manic-depressive illness, and particularly those in the throes of serious depression, were major targets for lobotomy. In fact, among the first 20 patients whom Moniz subjected to lobotomy, 9 were diagnosed with depression, 1 with mania, and 1 with manic-depressive illness. Moniz reported that 70 percent of these patients improved.[20] His results were widely disseminated, and lobotomy started to be used on an experimental basis through the 1930s. By the 1940s, lobotomy had taken off worldwide; by 1951, more than 18,000 had been performed in the United States alone. In 1949, Moniz received the Nobel Prize for his lobotomy discovery.

From its inception, lobotomy was mired in controversy. Many psychiatrists, neurologists, and neurosurgeons had grave misgivings about mucking about willy-nilly with the brain; it wasn't at all clear where the severed fibers were going, what they did, and how cutting them affected brain function. And lobotomy came with substantial side effects: apathy, socially inappropriate behavior, intellectual deterioration, and seizures among them. A well-known example of lobotomy's deleterious effects is the experience of Rosemary Kennedy, sister of President John Kennedy. In 1941, hoping that it would mitigate her troublesome behavior and violent mood swings, Joseph Kennedy, Rosemary's father, arranged for her to have a lobotomy. She was 23 years old. The procedure left her permanently incapacitated; after the lobotomy she could not walk or speak intelligibly, she was incontinent, and her mental capacity diminished to that of a 2-year-old. She required custodial care for the rest of her life.

Yet lobotomy did have some beneficial effects. It calmed some agitated patients, it relieved some patients of relentless obsessions and compulsions, and it could allay the anguish of severe depression. Perhaps what most accounted for its widespread use was that it made many patients with mental disorders more "manageable." As a result, some could leave the hospital and return to their homes. By the mid-1950s, the use of lobotomy started to decline. Its mixed and unpredictable results and its damaging side effects began to override its usefulness. Contributing most of all to lobotomy's demise was the introduction of psychiatric drugs, lithium among them, which calmed patients without putting them at risk for seizures and mental deterioration.

Even with the advent of lithium and, in the decades following its arrival, other effective treatments, manic-depressive illness remains a devastating condition. Not all people get better with treatment and a substantial minority do not use the prescribed medicine consistently or refuse it altogether; and even when treatment is helpful, people with manic-depressive illness remain subject to relapse. These relapses can have grave consequences. Periods of depression damage work and family life and come with unbearable hopelessness and despair. Today, about 6 percent of people with manic-depressive illness kill themselves, a rate of suicide 10 to 20 times greater than that of the general population. Although people in the throes of a manic episode often feel extraordinarily good, these episodes, with their frenzied activity and irrationality, wreak endless havoc, putting the victim at risk for legal and financial trouble and creating turmoil for their families.

Manic-depressive illness comes with other problems as well. People with this disorder have high rates of alcoholism and substance abuse. They are prone to early death and have twice the mortality rate of the general population. Some of this increased mortality can be attributed to suicide, but people with manic-depressive illness also have higher rates of death from natural causes, particularly diseases of the heart and blood vessels. The reasons for the increased physical vulnerability are not clear. The malnutrition and exhaustion that can be associated with both manic and depressive episodes may be partly to blame. Also at fault could be the difficulty that people with this disorder have in accessing medical care as well as following health recommendations.

The morbidity and mortality associated with manic-depressive illness certainly can diminish reproductive ability. Evolutionary theory suggests that the genes responsible for this illness should have been naturally selected against; under the pressures of natural selection, manic-depressive illness should have faded away. Yet the rates of this illness have remained high. So might the genes for manic-depressive illness confer some advantage that accounts for their persistence?

Maybe. A clue as to what that advantage might be comes from

studies of writers, poets, and artists. Conducted since the late nineteenth century, these studies have shown, with remarkable consistency, that manic-depressive illness is extraordinarily common in writers and artists—people who are creative. George Gordon (Lord Byron) was among the many eminent poets who suffered with the sustained extremes of mood and behavior characteristic of this disorder. Writing about his depression in a letter to a friend, he said, "I am so bilious—that I nearly lose my head—and so nervous that I cry for nothing—at least today I burst into tears all alone by myself over a cistern of gold fishes—which are not pathetic animals."[21] And commenting on the rage that typified his manic episodes, he said, "As long as I can remember anything, I recollect being subject to violent paroxysms of rage, so disproportioned to the cause, as to surprise me when they were over, and this still continues. I cannot coolly view anything that excites my feelings; and once the lurking devil in me is roused, I lose all command of myself."[22]

Manic-depressive illness is, in fact, most prevalent in poets; rates range from 20 to 40 percent. But the prevalence is also high (5 to 15 times greater than in the general population) in writers, artists, and composers.

It seems plausible that one or more of the genes that confer risk for manic-depressive illness also underlie creativity. It's not too much of a Darwinian stretch to say that the ability to think creatively improves one's chances of survival, to say nothing of the chances of finding a suitable mate. Can people who carry some of the manic-depressive genes or a "low dose" of these genes get the enhanced creativity without the illness? If so, that might explain, at least in part, the persistence of manic-depressive genes. A few studies have shown that the relatives of people with manic-depressive illness who are themselves psychiatrically normal score high on measures of creativity.[23] Thus, it appears that carriers of manic-depressive genes can, in fact, be especially creative without having the illness. For these people, manic-depressive genes may provide an evolutionary advantage that perhaps allows the genes and this illness to endure.

And endure it does. Since before antiquity to the present, it has afflicted millions. By the mid-twentieth century, although those who suffered from it were no longer chained to walls or operated on unnecessarily, manic depression was still a scourge that allowed no relief. The array of treatments applied to it, none of them save ECT offering any benefit and many of them dangerous, reflected both the gravity of the illness and the frustration of those attempting to heal it. In 1948, an unassuming young psychiatrist from a small country town in Australia stepped into this medical morass. What he happened upon restored the lives of people with manic-depressive illness and brought psychiatry into the scientific age.

2

The Naturalist

I N OCTOBER 1970, John Cade, president of the Australian and New Zealand College of Psychiatrists (ANZCP), gave his presidential address to the College. By then he had received worldwide recognition for his discovery that lithium can relieve mania. Toward the end of his address, he reminisced a bit about his career. "My own research efforts have been sporadic over many years," he said. "Most have ended in blind alleys. Some have been successful. All have been fun. In the process I have learned a great deal about the habits of termites, the length of snakes' tails, the meaning of the kookaburra's raucous cry, the length of the vagus nerve in the sleeping lizard, the eccentricities of lightning, the dermatological metamorphoses of chameleons, the ecology of my own garden, and en passant something of the causes and effective treatment of manic-depressive illness."[1]

Cade was not being facetious. Looking back near the end of his life, he said: "I have taken a tremendous intellectual pride in all discoveries I have made, irrespective of their importance or whether the same fact has been ascertained by others many times previously."[2] Indeed, his curiosity about the natural world and the satisfaction he got from his "discoveries" about it (not diminished at all by the fact that others had made the same discoveries) were, according to his friends and family—and by his own admission— among his foremost qualities. And the inventory of "discoveries" that he provided in his presidential address was far from a complete list. Cade was known for his interest in and knowledge of paw prints and most particularly for his expertise regarding scat— from all species. His son Peter recalls his father showing him the tiny six-sided pellets produced by the emperor gum moth caterpillar and explaining that from their shape one could deduce the six-sided structure of the caterpillar's anus.[3]

Although Cade clearly reveled in the recognition he eventually received for his lithium discovery and was gratified by its importance, he remarked on more than one occasion that his research on magpies brought him equal satisfaction. And to be sure, his investigation of magpies reflected, as much as any of his inquiries, both his intense curiosity and his confidence in plain, unfettered observation. White-backed magpies and black-backed magpies are both native to Australia. For much of the twentieth century, they were considered separate species, but Cade—and some professional ornithologists—wondered if they might be variants of one species. He decided to find out for himself, and in his presidential address he described how he went about it:

> With the utmost modesty, I should like to tell you of my greatest research, which took only four hours of careful observation to bring to a triumphant conclusion. It was designed to answer the simple question, "What is the relationship of the black-backed magpie to the white-backed?" Most would not regard the answer as likely to be fundamental to human happiness and might feel there are other more profitable investigations one might pursue. No doubt they would be correct, but

all the same the question had intrigued me for years. As you know, hereabouts they are all white-backed. . . . The black-backed bird breeds all the way up to Surfers Paradise, from north of the Great Dividing Range. Is he a separate species or an intra-species variant? Various zoologists I consulted from time to time did not seem to know. I discovered the answer by a careful roadside count when I drove one summer day from Wagga to West Brunswick. North of the Glenrowan Gap, they were all black backs. A few miles south of there, I saw my first white-back and several brindles with more black than white on the saddle. Going south, one found steadily more whites, and brindles with progressively more white than black. From Kilmore 60 miles south to Melbourne, it is an all-white population, but the immature young still had speckled white and grey saddles. Clearly therefore they are all intra-species variants.[4]

Apparently unknown to Cade—though it would not have dulled his enthusiasm for the research—an ornithologist had come to the same conclusion a few years earlier. This finding is now generally accepted as correct.

Cade's friends, colleagues, and family members—and Cade himself—would have agreed with his wife Jean when she summed up his life as "one of observation."[5] Moreover, Cade's inclination to thoroughly examine the world around him was a characteristic in short supply. Most of us see only what we expect to see. (As Yogi Berra supposedly put it: "If I didn't believe it, I wouldn't have seen it.") More troublesome, most of us ignore or fail to perceive the unexpected. But Cade seemed to have an aptitude for taking in the unforeseen. His son Jack recalls that the family was on a drive through the Black Forest when Cade suddenly announced that "he thought there were elephants up ahead in the forest."[6] There are, of course, no elephants in Australian forests and the family duly ridiculed his prediction. But then three elephants appeared at the side of the road. Cade had noticed a pile of dung on the side of the road too large to be from any other animal, and as it turned out, the circus was on tour.

Our consummate observer was born on August 18, 1912, in a small hospital in Horsham, Victoria, the major city in Australia's Wimmera area, about 190 miles northwest of Melbourne. The Cade family home was in Murtoa, a small country town about 20 miles from Horsham, where David Cade, John Cade's father, was the local general practitioner. Cade's mother, Ellen, a former nurse, and his two younger brothers, David and Frank, made up the rest of the family.

At the start of World War I, David Cade, already a veteran of the Boer War, enlisted at age 40 in the Australian Imperial Force (AIF), the Australian Army's expeditionary corps. He left Australia in 1915 and served as a medical officer with the 3rd Field Ambulance, a mobile medical unit, in Gallipoli and France. When he returned to Murtoa in 1919, he was a shattered man—demoralized, plagued with horrific memories, bereft of energy and vitality. He described himself as suffering from "war weariness." (Today his diagnosis would almost certainly be severe PTSD.) Perhaps in part because of his "war weariness," David Cade was a difficult father— remote, irritable, disinterested, austere.[7] He and his son John had a notably formal—stiff might be more accurate—relationship; John Cade never called his father anything but "Sir." Still, according to Cade's son Jack, John Cade "loved his father dearly."[8]

The demands of general practice, which included caring for the victims of the still raging flu pandemic, were more than David Cade could manage. Seeking a secure government salary and less demanding job, he sold his private practice and took a position as an asylum doctor in Victoria's Mental Hygiene Service. Over the next 25 years, David Cade served as the medical superintendent at several Victorian mental hospitals, and as was the custom of the time, the superintendent and his family lived in a house on the grounds of the asylum. As a result, John Cade grew up among people with severe mental illness. His son Jack feels that

John Cade's experience living on the grounds of these asylums had "a major bearing on his later deep understanding of the needs of the mentally ill."⁹

John Cade got his secondary school education at Melbourne's prestigious Scotch College (it boasts more notable Australians among its alumni than any other school in the country). In 1929, he went on to study medicine at the University of Melbourne and graduated at age 21 with honors in all subjects. In his last year of medical school, he picked up the forensics medicine prize for receiving the highest grade in the forensics examination.

Cade was born left-handed, but as was the custom at the time, his teachers forced him to write with his right hand. He ended up playing golf and tennis with both hands and was proficient at both. His son Jack recalled that "he could play a round of nine holes of golf after an absence of many years and, armed with only a 5 iron and putter, return a score in the low 40s. His sons were never able to beat him at golf or even tennis at least until after the first set and then only when he was much older."¹⁰ As a boy, Cade learned the rudiments of boxing from one of the asylum patients and developed some proficiency in this sport as well; at university he boxed against fellow students who also were adept in the ring.

After graduating from medical school, Cade served for one year as a house officer (resident) at Melbourne's St Vincent's Hospital and then decided to study pediatrics. In 1936, he started his residency at the Royal Children's Hospital in Melbourne. Soon after, he developed a severe case of bilateral pneumonia. Gravely ill, he was confined to bed at the Children's Hospital. This was in the pre-antibiotic era, and Cade came close to dying; a priest was called. But he pulled through, and there was an upside to this nearly tragic event. One of the nurses caring for Cade was a fetching brunette named Estana Evelyn Jean Charles (everyone called her Jean). The day he was discharged, Cade came back and asked her out to dinner.¹¹ They were married the following year and remained so until Cade's death in 1980.

At some point in 1936, Cade decided that pediatrics was not

for him. He opted for psychiatry and, following in his father's footsteps, joined the Victorian Department of Mental Hygiene. In late 1936, he was appointed as a medical officer and headed for Beechworth Mental Hospital, where his father had worked and the family had lived 15 years earlier.

At Beechworth, Cade, 24 years old and a newly minted doctor, began his psychiatric research career. Cade often denigrated his research credentials and his methods; he repeatedly portrayed himself as an "enthusiastic amateur" and famously said after he had achieved renown for his lithium discovery, "I am not a scientist. I am only an old prospector who happened to pick up a nugget."[12] Still, early in his career he showed a penchant for investigation. Moreover, he believed that psychiatrists have an obligation to carry out research. In 1951, concluding a prestigious Beattie-Smith Lecture at the University of Melbourne, Cade said:

> Let each one of us engaged in the treatment of mental illness deliberately set out to investigate for ourselves some one of the numerous problems which arise, according to our own particular training or enthusiasm. Let us never rest content with the present bounds of knowledge. It is for us to initiate a particular approach to a psychiatric problem, and if we have not the necessary knowledge or technical training—if, for example, it involves a specialized knowledge of biochemistry or physiology—then let us cultivate and coopt our colleagues in those specialties.[13]

And nearly 20 years later, in his presidential address to the ANZCP, Cade continued to exhort his colleagues: "Almost everyone can and should do research, both because almost everyone has an unique observational opportunity at some time in his life which he has an obligation to record, and also because the intellectual discipline and technical training that it imposes is an essential prerequisite to expertise in a professional field."[14]

It didn't take Cade long to come upon an "observational opportunity." An attendant at Beechworth drew his attention to extensive bruising in a number of patients. Cade wondered if unnecessary force inflicted by staff or assaults by other patients were to blame. Although not implausible, these didn't seem adequate explanations. So Cade looked elsewhere, and he soon found the answer. Aware that easy bruising is a sign of scurvy, a condition resulting from inadequate vitamin C, Cade tested these patients' vitamin C levels. Their levels were "grossly deficient." Cade went on to conduct a survey of patients' nutritional status at Beechworth and at Mont Park Mental Hospital, where his father was medical superintendent. It turned out that inadequate levels of vitamin C—and scurvy—were rampant among the residents of both hospitals. It didn't take much sleuthing for him to pinpoint the problem. Although the hospital gardens produced loads of fresh fruits and vegetables (a good source of vitamin C), the patients, even those who harvested the crops, did not eat the produce fresh. As Cade put it: "All the produce was taken to the hospital kitchen and thrown into the huge copper cauldrons where every thermolabile vitamin, and especially ascorbic acid (Vitamin C), was very thoroughly exterminated."[15] He sent a report of his findings to the Director of Mental Hygiene. Among other things, he recommended that the patients' diet include fresh fruits and vegetables. His suggestion was implemented throughout the mental hospitals in Victoria. Further, his report prompted the department to appoint its first dietitian. Vitamin deficiencies in Victorian mental hospitals became a thing of the past.

Cade began to research and write scientific papers at a relatively young age; his first published paper depicted a Beechworth patient who in 1938 died, it seemed, as a result of widespread spasm of her arteries. Reporting on this patient in the July 30, 1938, issue of the *Medical Journal of Australia*, Cade provided detailed findings from her autopsy and questioned whether her unique mode of death may have been a consequence of reflex arterial changes following the presence of a large gallstone in her intestine.

In mid-1939, Cade got a taste of sophisticated research. By that time he had moved to the department's Bundoora Repatriation Mental Hospital. A flu outbreak had hit the hospital, and Cade worked with Frank Burnet, an eminent virologist and immunologist, on a study measuring antibodies in afflicted patients. Burnet went on to win a Nobel Prize and become Australia's most renowned scientist. The paper reporting their study appeared in 1940 in the *Medical Journal of Australia*, with Cade as coauthor.[16]

At around the same time, Cade surveyed the patients in Victoria's mental hospitals who had a diagnosis of primary dementia (now called schizophrenia) and examined differences between men and women in the age at which the disease began. He wrote, on his own, a brief paper reporting his findings: "A Statistical Study of the Onset of Primary Dementia." It, too, appeared in 1940 in the *Medical Journal of Australia*.

So, as a junior medical officer, in addition to looking after patients, Cade did a bit of research and got a start on scientific writing. He also studied for his doctor of medicine (MD) degree. At that time in Australia, the MD was a postgraduate medical degree, analogous to a PhD, meant for doctors aspiring to scientific investigation. Typically, the medical school graduates who did this additional schooling were headed for careers in research. The degree required either a thesis or passing a comprehensive examination. Cade went the examination route. The University of Melbourne provided an extensive reading list and advanced courses. Candidates for the degree were expected to be knowledgeable, and were examined in both basic sciences and the gamut of clinical medicine. Cade's examinations included physiology, pathology, immunology, and clinical medicine, including the history of medicine. He got his MD in 1938.

By the beginning of 1940, Cade had done some research, had cut his teeth on those early articles, and had his MD in hand. He was ready—and eager—to come up with some fresh approaches to the problems besetting his chosen field. Nevertheless, more than five years would pass, five "interminable years," as Cade put it, before he could devote himself to a research project.

On September 3, 1939, Australia had declared war on Germany. Soon after, the 2nd Australian Imperial Force began to mobilize. Cade, again following in his father's footsteps, enlisted in the AIF and in July 1940 was posted to the 2nd/9th Field Ambulance as a captain.

Cade was no stranger to the military. As a university student and at his father's urging, he had joined the Melbourne University Rifles, a military training group for students. In 1935, soon after graduation, he had volunteered for the Militia, the Australian Army Reserve.

Cade spent the last months of 1940 in military training, and in February 1941 he left Sydney for the British colony of Malaya (today, independent Malaysia), sailing on the *Queen Mary*, the former luxury liner now refitted as a troop ship. Although Cade was a trained psychiatrist, his position in the AIF was that of a general medical officer. There were, in fact, no psychiatrists for either the Australian or British troops on Malaya, who eventually numbered almost 150,000.

This was not a simple oversight. Senior medical officers at Australian Army Headquarters didn't believe, initially, that psychiatrists had skills that could be useful near the battlefield. They relied on junior general medical officers to "detect the malingerer and bash back the neurotic," and they feared that "over-enthusiastic psychiatrists might start a landslide which might sweep away a goodly proportion of the essential manpower through a broadened channel leading to the way out."[17]

Churchill expressed the prevailing view at that time—at least in the Commonwealth—on the role of psychiatry in the military: "It would be sensible to restrict as much as possible the work of these gentlemen, who are capable of doing an immense amount of harm with what may very easily degenerate into charlatanry. The tightest hand should be kept over them and they should not be allowed to quarter themselves upon the Fighting services at the public expense." Churchill did allow that "there are, no doubt, easily recognizable cases which may benefit from treatment of this kind," but went on to insist that "it is very wrong to disturb large numbers of healthy, normal men and women by asking the kind of odd questions in which the psychiatrists specialize. There are quite enough hangers-on and camp followers already."[18]

So Cade, alongside the men of the 9th Field Ambulance, looked after the general health needs of the Australian soldiers. The 8th division of the AIF, which included Cade's unit, had come to Malaya to help the British garrison defend the Malay Peninsula and the island of Singapore from an expected Japanese attack. Cade landed in Malaya on February 15, and for the next nine months, although life was less than pleasant and the heat and humidity oppressive, things were quiet, camaraderie was plentiful, and the unfamiliar, exotic environment held some interest. Cade treated soldiers for everything from fungal infections and dysentery to venereal disease. He also culled and sent home more than a few men who were unfit for duty on medical or psychological grounds. In September 1941, Cade was promoted to major. His interest and skills in psychiatry earned him the nickname Mad Major, and it stuck with him for the rest of the war.

On December 8, 1941 (local time), about 50 minutes before they attacked Pearl Harbor, the Japanese invaded Malaya, landing troops from its 25th Army on Malaya's northeast coast. The campaign that ensued pitted the Japanese against the British Commonwealth forces—British, Australian, and Indian units—ensconced on Malaya. It went on for two months, was the first major battle of the Pacific War, and ended in disaster for the defenders.

The Commonwealth forces outnumbered the Japanese 2 to 1 (140, 000 to 70,000), but in all other ways the Japanese had the clear advantage; they enjoyed far superior air and naval power, and their soldiers were thoroughly trained and often battle-hardened, many having fought in China, whereas the Commonwealth soldiers were by and large inexperienced (some of the Australian reinforcements set out for combat after only two weeks of training). The Japanese had 200 tanks, the Commonwealth none. The Japanese used bicycles, allowing their troops to carry more equipment and move quickly on paths through the thick jungle terrain—territory that the Allies believed impassable. (The Japanese had not brought bicycles with them, but they knew from their intelligence that bikes were plentiful in Malaya and confiscated them from civilians and retailers.) The Japanese commanders made few false moves, whereas the Commonwealth commanders made one tactical blunder after another, to some extent a result of overestimating Japanese troop strength and underestimating their own capabilities.

During December and January, the Japanese army, supported by air and naval forces, advanced rapidly and steadily down the Malay Peninsula, killing, wounding, capturing, and sometimes torturing scores of Allied soldiers. When the invasion started, Cade, stationed in the south of the peninsula, was at some distance from the battle zone. But as the Allied forces retreated toward Singapore, Cade was in the midst of the debacle. As the battle raged, his capacity for keen observation and cool-headedness served him well. In an episode that took on mythic status in the annals of the 2nd/9th Field Ambulance, Cade was riding at night in the front seat of an army truck when he spotted Japanese soldiers on the side of the road some distance away. Without mentioning what he had seen, he simply instructed the driver to turn around, which the driver did, saving the lives of all the men involved. When later the driver asked him, "Why didn't you tell me?" Cade replied, "I wasn't sure what your reaction would be."[19]

By the end of January 1942, Malaya was lost and the Commonwealth forces had withdrawn to Singapore for one last stand. They blew a hole in the causeway connecting Malaya to Singapore and prepared to defend the island. On February 8, following days of intense aerial and artillery bombardment, the Japanese forces invaded Singapore. The ensuing battle went on for a week. Allied forces were exhausted and demoralized. Their water supply was uncertain, food was running low, and they had no aircraft and little ammunition. Despite the fact that the Allies outnumbered the Japanese 85,000 to 30,000, they had no prospect of prevailing. Nonetheless, Churchill insisted that they fight on. He cabled General Archibald Wavell, commander of Allied forces in Southeast Asia, on the evening of February 10:

> I think you ought to realise the way we view the situation in Singapore. It was reported to the Cabinet by the C.I.G.S. [Chief of the Imperial General Staff] that Percival [commander of Allied forces on Malaya and Singapore] has over 100,000 men . . . It is doubtful whether the Japanese have as many in the whole Malay peninsula . . . In these circumstances the defenders must greatly outnumber Japanese forces who have crossed the straits, and in a well-contested battle they should destroy them. There must at this stage be no thought of saving the troops or sparing the population. The battle must be fought to the bitter end at all costs. The 18th Division has a chance to make its name in history. Commanders and senior officers should die with their troops. The honour of the British Empire and of the British Army is at stake. I rely on you to show no mercy to weakness in any form. With the Russians fighting as they are and the Americans so stubborn at Luzon, the whole reputation of our country and our race is involved. It is expected that every unit will be brought into close contact with the enemy and fight it out.[20]

Wavell ordered General Percival to continue the fight, and the Allies did continue to put up some resistance. But they had lost critical facilities, including water reservoirs, airfields, and supply depots, and without sufficient resources to continue the battle, they were facing a massive slaughter of both troops and civilians. On February 15, they surrendered. Churchill called it the "worst disaster" in British military history.

The Japanese had not expected to prevail so completely (they knew they were outnumbered), and they didn't at first have the resources to manage the roughly 50,000 soldiers (about 35,000 Brits and 15,000 Australians) who were now their prisoners. On a peninsula known as Changi, jutting out from the east end of

Singapore Island, stood Changi Prison, a facility for civilian criminals, and near the prison were several barracks that had housed the British garrison. On February 17, 1942, the Japanese herded their prisoners to these barracks, which were thereafter referred to as the Changi prisoner of war camp, or simply Changi. The Australians ended up in the Selarang Barracks, with many of the British in Roberts Barracks. Cade and the men of the 2nd/9th Field Ambulance were among the first to enter Changi.

At first, the POWs were left largely to their own devices; they were free to roam around the area, and guards rarely appeared. But over the following months, the Japanese tightened security, built fences around individual camps, and restricted movement between them.

A hospital to care for the sick and wounded was a first priority. Initially, the British and Australian medical officers set up separate hospitals; Cade and his fellow medical officers had charge of a 270-bed facility. Within a month, the Japanese decided that the POWs should have a combined hospital under one commanding officer. Accordingly, a portion of Roberts Barracks was reborn as Roberts Hospital. The Australian and British officers agreed that medical care should be segregated, with Australians treating Australians and British treating British. So although it was one hospital, Roberts contained separate wards for Australian and British POWs.

The hospital held 2,500 patients, and it was Cade's professional home. He worked as a general medical officer, but as the doctor most qualified to handle psychiatric matters, he also managed the joint British and Australian psychiatric ward, one of the few joint services. It was composed of 10 to 12 beds and housed the small number of POWs who became blatantly disturbed. Both Australian and British doctors called on Cade when they needed psychiatric consultation.[21]

Changi was in some ways an unusual Japanese POW camp. The ultimate death toll of 850 men was substantially lower than that at other Japanese POW camps, where the average death rate was 27 percent. The POWs at Changi did not escape Japanese brutality, but summary executions, beatings, and torture were relatively rare. The Australian and British officers pretty much ran the place, military discipline remained intact, and contact with the Japanese captors was, with the exception of work parties, a matter for the senior officers. The POWs were initially quite demoralized—they felt betrayed by their commanders and had not expected to surrender and become prisoners. But as time went on, a complex community took root, and all sorts of recreational and educational activities proliferated: theatrical performances, concerts, sporting events, lectures. A body called the Changi Medical Society even held monthly meetings. Morale improved and, given the circumstances, remained surprisingly good.

Nonetheless, Changi's notoriety is well deserved. Throughout its three-and-a-half-year existence, it served as a source of workers for the Japanese empire. Thousands of Changi POWs were shipped to labor camps in Borneo and Japan, to the infamous Burma-Thailand railway and elsewhere, to work under brutal conditions—and often to perish. All his life Cade was troubled by the fact that, believing the fresh air and activity might help them, he sent about 100 of his patients to the Burma-Thailand railway, all of whom died as a result of the move.

There was a continuous flow of prisoners in and out of Changi. For those interned there, the biggest problem was malnutrition. The rations provided by the Japanese were grossly inadequate with respect to both total calories and essential nutrients. The 1929 Geneva Convention stipulated that POWs were to receive humane treatment, including sufficient food, but the Japanese did not consider themselves bound by the convention; their government had signed but not ratified it. Furthermore, the Japanese believed that surrender was dishonorable, unthinkable actually; soldiers were supposed to fight to the death. Accordingly, they regarded the POWs as beneath contempt and they starved them with impunity.

The rations provided by the Japanese consisted of a portion of polished rice each day, with a small amount of meat occasionally added. On this regimen it didn't take long for deficiency diseases to make their way through the camps. Most worrisome, because it could result in heart failure and death, was beriberi, but thousands of POWs suffered other ill effects of vitamin deficiency, including pellagra, stomatitis (inflammation of the mouth and lips), painful feet, rashes of all sorts, and impaired vision.

The POWs did everything they could to supplement their food rations. They started vegetable gardens, work parties pilfered food from supply ships, and they bartered for food with local merchants. They also formed a nutrition advisory committee that included experts on the biochemistry of nutrition and doctors experienced in deficiency diseases. The committee surveyed the nutritional value of the available food, came up with several concoctions designed to provide essential vitamins, particularly the B vitamins necessary to heal and prevent deficiency diseases, and then went on to investigate, in controlled research studies, the relative benefits of these concoctions—rice polishings, yeast, and grass soup among them. The grass soup—rich in riboflavin—was a testament to the POWs' ingenuity. Using scythes and reaping hooks that they had designed and made themselves, the POWs cut tons of grass and leaves. They put the cuttings into a device constructed by the engineers that thoroughly shredded them and extracted a liquid. It was light orange, bitter, and tasted awful; the men called it Tiger's Piss. But it was a good treatment for stomatitis and prevented that and other deficiency diseases. With the improvement in nutrition, the incidence of deficiency diseases went down, but there was simply never enough food; the POWs continued to be hungry and malnourished and to suffer weight loss, debility, and emaciation.

Cade was by all accounts an exemplary medical officer. The men who served with him admired—indeed, treasured—him for his medical and psychiatric competence and for his equanimity, resilience, and courage. He was one of the men who delivered the BBC daily news bulletin known as the "Canary." The POWs were not permitted to have radios, but there were a number hidden around the camps. Cade would listen to the BBC news, make notes of the broadcasts, and then deliver the news to an audience of POWs, mimicking a news broadcaster. When it seemed too dangerous to carry written reports (Cade risked severe punishment if he was discovered carrying such reports), he committed the entire update to memory and delivered it verbatim to his audience. Years later, recalling Cade's recitals of the forbidden BBC news, Cade's men described his manner of delivery "as if he were in front of the BBC microphone."[22]

During his captivity, Cade seemed to solidify some of his notions about psychiatric illness, particularly the idea that severe psychiatric disorders have a physical basis. He noted that whereas many of the POWs were demoralized and distressed, very few had the unremitting despair and immobility of classic melancholia. Cade figured that something in addition to the appalling circumstances must be causing the melancholia. Further, when he conducted autopsies on patients with psychiatric illness who had died, he noted brain abnormalities like tumors and blood clots. Looking back on the years at Changi, Cade said: " I could see that so many of the psychiatric patients suffering from the so-called functional psychoses appeared to be sick people in the medical sense. This fired my ambition to discover their etiology."[23]

On September 5, 1945, troops of the 5th Indian Division liberated Changi. Cade left Singapore on September 23, sailing for home on the SS *Largs Bay*. Launched as a mixed passenger/cargo ship in 1921, the SS *Largs Bay* served as a troop transport during World War II. Not as grand as the *Queen Mary*, which had brought Cade to Singapore four and a half years earlier, it nevertheless served the purpose. It reached Darwin, on Australia's north coast, on September 29 and arrived in Sydney, its final destination, on October 9.

After being interned at Changi for three and a half years, Cade was suffering from severe malnutrition. But he was raring to get back to work long before the ship ferrying him home reached the dock. En route, on September 26, Cade wrote, in a letter to Jean: "The old brain box is simmering with ideas. I believe this long period of waiting has allowed many of my notions in psychiatry to crystallize, and I'm just bursting to put them to the test. If they work out, they would represent a great advance in the knowledge of manic-depressive insanity and primary dementia—sounds like my usual over-optimism, doesn't it? Well there is only one way to find out—test it and see."[24]

3

Lithium

LITHIUM HAS been around for a long time. It was one of the first three elements, along with helium and hydrogen, produced by the Big Bang. So it has been with us forever or, more precisely, for nearly 14 billion years. It's the lightest metal, and like the closely related sodium, it's an alkali, readily forming salts when mixed with acids. Like lye and other alkaline substances, lithium compounds can be caustic and slimy; they are an important constituent of grease.

Because lithium is a highly reactive element, promptly bonding with other substances in air, water, and elsewhere, it never occurs freely in nature but rather in combination with other elements as salts such as lithium carbonate and lithium chloride. Many lithium salts, like the lithium carbonate used as a treatment for bipolar disorder, look like ordinary table salt. When purified in the laboratory, lithium is a silvery white metal about the density of pine wood. It cuts easily, like butter, with a kitchen knife.

Although lithium occurs throughout the earth's surface, particularly in rocks, mineral springs, and seawater, and in trace amounts in plants and animals, it was not identified as a discrete element until the early nineteenth century. José Bonifácio de Andrada e Silva, a Brazilian statesman, naturalist, and poet, set the stage for the detection of lithium when in 1800 he discovered a new mineral in rocks extracted from an iron mine on the Swedish island of Uto. He named the new mineral petalite. Nothing more was heard of petalite until 1817, when once again it was found on Uto, this time by Eric Thomas Svedenstjerna, a Swedish mettalurgist. Svedenstjerna sent samples of petalite to various acquaintances. Some of it ended up in the laboratory of Jöns Jacob Berzelius, the foremost Swedish chemist of the day. Berzelius handed over the petalite to his young assistant, Johan August Arfwedson, who proceeded to analyze it. Arfwedson found that 96 percent of the petalite consisted of alumina and silica. The remaining 4 percent was an alkaline substance that did not respond to the usual tests for known alkaline elements. Arfwedson concluded, correctly, that he had discovered a new element, and in light of the fact that it had been found in a rock, Berzelius suggested the name lithium after the Greek word *lithos*, meaning stone.

Over the ensuing decades, other chemists went on to purify lithium, extracting it from its salts, and to characterize the properties of lithium and its compounds. By the mid-twentieth century, lithium had begun to find its way into commercial use. Today it has a number of important industrial applications. Because it is both light and a good conductor of electricity, lithium makes up the batteries that power pacemakers, mobile phones, and other small electronic devices. Stable over a wide temperature range, it is an important constituent of ceramics and glass, and it is used in a high-temperature grease in aircraft and other engines. Lithium is highly hygroscopic (it attracts and absorbs water), rendering it a key component of industrial drying systems and air conditioners. And when lithium is alloyed with aluminum and other metals, it results in a material that is both lightweight and strong, a vital component of aircraft, bicycles, and trains. Lithium is also an essential ingredient of hydrogen bombs and nuclear reactors.

Although today lithium is an important treatment for bipolar illness, its use as a treatment accounts for a miniscule proportion of its applications. But for the first 100 years after its discovery, lithium's only use was as a medical treatment.

In the mid-nineteenth century, just a few decades after chemists first isolated and characterized lithium, several medical practitioners noted that lithium compounds could dissolve uric acid. Lithium did this by joining with uric acid to form lithium urate, a soluble salt. This observation launched lithium's introduction into medicine. At the time, prominent doctors believed that excess uric acid was the culprit behind a good many ills. So based on its ability to dissolve uric acid, physicians of the mid-nineteenth century began using lithium to treat a wide range of ailments, including headaches, diabetes, asthma, indigestion, obesity, skin disorders, rheumatism, and—more than 50 years before Cade made his groundbreaking discovery—an assortment of psychiatric conditions. Uric acid, in fact, continuously pokes its head into the lithium story.

It is possible that John Cade drew some of his inspiration for giving lithium to manic patients from the much earlier use of lithium in some medical and psychiatric conditions, including depression. In all likelihood, Cade selected the doses of lithium that he first gave to manic patients based on the doses that his predecessors had given to people suffering ailments presumably caused by uric acid. What's more, as we shall see, the experiments that Cade did with guinea pigs, which allowed him to detect lithium's psychological properties, rested on lithium's knack for combining with uric acid to form lithium urate. So uric acid, an ordinary and for the most part insignificant constituent of body fluids, is a thread that joins some of the main elements of the lithium story.

Uric acid is a breakdown product of purines, biological molecules that are essential components of DNA, enzymes, and other key bits of cells. For the most part, uric acid minds its own business, floating about harmlessly until the kidneys get rid of it. The exception to this humdrum picture is gout. When uric acid gets abnormally high—as can happen when one eats large amounts of purine-rich foods (some meats and fish) and in rare instances when the kidneys can't properly dispose of it—the uric acid produces crystals that wind up in joints. These uric acid crystals create the excruciating joint pain typical of gout. High uric acid can also give rise to kidney stones.

Alexander Lipowitz, a German chemist who had his hand in everything from cement manufacture to photography, got the lithium/uric acid ball rolling in 1841, when he pulverized some lepidolite, an ore containing lithium, mixed it in boiling water with the barely soluble uric acid, and found that he had produced the far more soluble lithium urate. Two years later, Alexander Ure, a British surgeon, took the step that started lithium on its journey as a medical treatment, a journey that a century later brought lithium to John Cade's makeshift laboratory.

Ure had a particular interest in finding a remedy for gout and for the urinary stones that often accompany it. Part of his motivation may have come from the fact that his father, an eminent scientist, had suffered with this disease for many years. Ure had experimented with chemical methods for dissolving gouty stones, many of which contain large amounts of uric acid. Encouraged by Lipowitz's observation that lithium could dissolve uric acid, Ure placed a sizable bladder stone, composed largely of uric acid, in a solution of lithium carbonate. Five hours later much of the stone had melted away. As Ure pointed out in the paper that he read to the Pharmaceutical Society describing this experiment, his observation suggested that injecting lithium carbonate directly into the bladder might be a good way of reducing the size of bladder stones. The only thing that had stopped him from trying this as a treatment, he said, was the scarcity of lithium carbonate. He ended his comments by putting in a plug for pharmaceutical chemists to begin getting enough lithium carbonate ready for clinical use.

Ure's appeal for more lithium carbonate largely fell on deaf ears, and it wasn't until 1859, 16 years later, that he was able to get his hands on enough lithium carbonate to try it as a treatment. His patient was a 56-year-old man with a large and uncomfortable bladder stone. Ure believed that the stone consisted chiefly of uric acid, which turned out to be the case, and proceeded to inject a solution of lithium carbonate into the bladder. He did this every other day or so for several weeks. Disappointingly, the stone refused to get smaller. To "expedite matters," Ure resorted to crushing the stone with a lithotrite, an instrument inserted into the bladder. After doing this a number of times, he had broken up much of the stone and a successful conclusion seemed likely. Unfortunately, before Ure got rid of the final fragments of stone, the patient died. The report of this case appeared in the August 25, 1860, issue of the eminent British medical journal *The Lancet*. The report did not mention the cause of death. It did make clear, though, that despite lithium carbonate's failure to dissolve the stone, Ure was not ready to give up on lithium. It seemed, he wrote, that "the solvent had in some measure lessened the cohesion of the concretion and increased its friability."[1]

By this time, however, whether or not lithium could dissolve bladder stones was largely beside the point. Sir Alfred Baring Garrod, a prominent British physician and contemporary of Ure, had cooked up a far larger medical role for lithium. Garrod was familiar with Ure's bladder stone work and had repeated his original experiment, but with a gouty bone instead of a bladder stone. He placed a finger bone, which featured a prominent gouty (uric acid) deposit at the joint, in a solution of lithium carbonate. Within several days, the deposit had disappeared.

Garrod went on to propose, in an influential series of books, that gout was a result of excess uric acid and that lithium carbonate, because it could dissolve uric acid, was a valuable remedy. But Garrod didn't stop there. He propagated the notion that excess uric acid was behind an assortment of other afflictions, from headaches to diabetes to a wide range of mental disturbances. This concept, known as the "uric acid diathesis" (a tendency to produce too much uric acid), captivated the medical profession. By the end of the nineteenth century, influential physicians throughout Europe and the United States had embraced the concept. By this time, medical authorities had included an amazing variety of diseases in the uric acid diathesis—everything from heart disease to intestinal ailments to asthma to tuberculosis. Any of these diseases, presumed to result from excess uric acid, was a candidate for treatment with lithium. Now widely available as a result of Garrod's recommendations, lithium became a regular part of the doctor's tool kit.

The uric acid diathesis remained a leading theory about the cause of disease well into the twentieth century, and it's easy to understand why. Given the fact that gout was associated with high uric acid and that people with gout sometimes suffered from other conditions as well, it was not implausible that uric acid contributed to these other conditions. Furthermore, the notion that a single culprit could be behind so many diseases has intuitive appeal. It's a notion that has been with us since the humoral theories of antiquity, through the disturbances of vital forces central to traditional Chinese and Ayurvedic medicine, to some contemporary views. Today, many people believe that spinal misalignment causes all sorts of disorders, that "stress" is the source of innumerable maladies, and that eating organic fruits and vegetables will prevent everything from heart disease to cancer.

Although it was clear from Ure's and Garrod's experiments that a lithium solution could dissolve uric acid in a test tube, it was not at all clear that lithium would have an effect on uric acid in the body. Nonetheless, Garrod advised that lithium carbonate be taken orally as a treatment for gout and other uric acid diathesis conditions. Lithium, he thought, would dissolve the circulating uric acid. More uric acid would come out in the urine, and the high uric acid levels would come down to normal. Garrod and others managed to convince themselves that at least some people with uric acid diathesis conditions showed signs of excess uric acid—such as uric acid crystals or high concentrations of uric acid in their urine (also seen in normal urine)—and that lithium carbonate improved some of the symptoms of gout and other conditions. Along with its intuitive appeal, the uric acid diathesis concept brought with it a seemingly rational treatment, a boon in an era when there were few effective treatments for anything.

Later studies eventually showed that lithium taken by mouth has no effect on uric acid or its elimination, partly because other compounds circulating in the body interfere with lithium's dissolving ability. Moreover, in the early decades of the twentieth century, it gradually became clear that uric acid is not, in fact, the cause of the many diseases attributed to it. Accordingly, lithium carbonate started to lose its appeal as a universal remedy. Further, as systematic observation and other features of scientific medicine began to take precedence over intuition and the pronouncements of authorities, lithium's lack of effect on the countless uric acid diseases became apparent. By the mid-twentieth century, the medical establishment had discarded the uric acid diathesis and dispensed with lithium as a credible treatment for anything.

But in the nineteenthth century, doctors regularly subjected their patients to bloodletting and purging and treated them with a hodgepodge of tonics and concoctions, despite the absence of any real evidence that these therapies provided benefit. Likewise, they remained undeterred by the lack of firm evidence for lithium carbonate's value. Physicians prescribed lithium for an assortment of medical conditions well into the twentiethth century, when its lack of effect became irrefutable.

One of the nineteenth-century doctors who jumped on the uric acid/lithium bandwagon was the Danish physician Carl Lange. Lange is best known for being one of the originators, along with the American psychologist William James, of the still influential James–Lange theory of emotion. This theory proposes, somewhat counterintuitively, that emotions don't produce physical changes but rather that physical changes produce emotions. According to James and Lange, when you come upon a bear and your heart rate goes up and you become tremulous, it is not that fear gives rise to these responses but rather that the perception of these physical responses gives rise to the emotion of fear. Simply stated, you don't run because you're afraid; you're afraid because you run. Lange's discourse on emotion was widely translated and brought him international renown.

But Lange had more than one string in his bow. In 1886, the year after he published his work on emotion, he came out with a treatise on what he called periodical depressions. In it he described a series of patients he had cared for in his medical practice who had repeated depressions of milder severity than is usually seen by psychiatrists. He noticed what he thought was an unusual sediment in these patients' urine and assumed, incorrectly, that the sediment was uric acid. Lange went on to hypothesize that these depressions were caused by excess uric acid and suggested that they could be treated and prevented by the conventional (at the time) therapies for uric acid conditions, which included lithium carbonate. In later writings he explicitly mentioned lithium carbonate as a treatment for these uric acid depressions. The lithium doses he advised were comparable to those used today for bipolar illness, and Lange reported favorable outcomes with this regimen.

Lange's colleagues in Denmark knew of his work, but for the most part the larger psychiatric community did not learn of it. Part of the reason for this lack of recognition was that Lange wrote his treatise in Danish, and it was translated only into German— and that not until 10 years later. (It got an English translation in 2001.) Although psychiatrists in Denmark came to regard Lange's description of periodic depression as an important and long-lasting contribution to psychiatric classification, they discounted his ideas about lithium treatment. And it's not hard to understand why.

Soon after Lange came out with his treatment for depression, the uric acid diathesis started to lose credibility. Given that the rationale for prescribing lithium had rested on the now discredited belief that uric acid causes the depression, psychiatrists discounted any role for lithium in the treatment of this illness.

Today, however, lithium carbonate is in fact recognized as a valuable treatment for recurrent depression, and specifically for the *prevention* of recurrent depression, just as Lange suggested. Some credit Lange with being the first to use lithium for this condition or, for that matter, to use lithium explicitly and systematically for any psychiatric condition. Ironically, because Lange proposed lithium treatment for the wrong reason (uric acid), its usefulness was disregarded; more than 60 years passed before John Cade rediscovered it.

Before we close the book on Carl Lange, his younger brother Fritz (Frederick) deserves mention. Fritz was a psychiatrist in charge of a Danish asylum, and taking his lead from Carl, he treated several hundred acutely depressed patients with lithium carbonate. In 1894, he reported that these patients improved within a few days to several weeks of getting lithium. After a brief spurt of attention, Fritz's work with lithium and depression, like that of his brother, was ignored and eventually forgotten.

Although Carl and Fritz Lange may have been the first to formally propose lithium as a treatment for a psychiatric condition—and, in support of their claims, to provide plentiful and detailed observations of patients—both before and after their seminal work, other late nineteenth-century physicians had in fact theorized about lithium's potential as a remedy for psychiatric afflictions. Garrod and other advocates of the uric acid diathesis believed that mental symptoms commonly went along with gout and excess uric acid. They thought that uric acid attacked the brain and as a result caused all sorts of mental derangements, including melancholy and, as Garrod put it, "gouty mania." Garrod and others treated all signs of the uric acid diathesis with lithium compounds and reported that along with other symptoms, mental ones improved as well.

Quite apart from the uric acid diathesis, in 1870, Silas Weir Mitchell, the eminent American neurologist, proposed lithium bromide as a treatment for epilepsy. It worked fairly well, probably because bromine is a good sedative, and it continued as an epilepsy treatment well into the twentieth century. Mitchell also gave lithium bromide to people with an assortment of nervous symptoms, some of whom were probably suffering from depression, and reported that they got relief. Again, the relief may have come from the bromine portion of the compound, not the lithium.

The work that seems to most directly foreshadow Cade's discovery came from William Hammond, a professor of nervous and mental diseases at New York's Bellevue Hospital. In his 1871 textbook on diseases of the nervous system, Hammond reported that he had used lithium bromide to treat patients with acute mania and found that it swiftly and effectively calmed them.[2] Hammond used exceptionally high doses, and it's not clear if it was the lithium or bromine portion of the compound that produced the results. In his later textbooks, published in 1882, 1883, and 1890, Hammond did not mention the use of lithium.

In the last decades of the nineteenth century and well into the twentieth, in parallel with the emergence of the uric acid diathesis and the belief that lithium was its key treatment, lithium enjoyed public acclaim as a first-rate cure-all in the form of "lithia water," bottled mineral water featuring lithium. Part of the enthusiasm for lithium came from, and was supported by, the uric acid diathesis, but by the late nineteenth century, lithium had taken on a life of its own as the remedy for all our ills.

Lithium historians trace the enthusiasm for lithium water to the mineral baths and springs treasured as a cure since antiquity. Soranus of Ephesus, the Greek physician of the second century CE, recommended alkaline mineral water as a remedy for all sorts of things, including mania. Through the ensuing centuries, physicians continued to recommend mineral baths for a wide range of afflictions, and people visited the baths both for treatment and recreation.

By the mid-nineteenth century, not long after its discovery, lithium turned up as one of the ingredients of mineral springs. With the advent of the uric acid diathesis as the explanation for an assortment of ills and the widespread application of lithium as its treatment, the promotion of mineral waters now had a "scientific rationale." Their popularity boomed. By the last decade of the nineteenth century, people were flocking to mineral springs and the resorts that sprang up around them. Some of these springs contained trace amounts of lithium and some no lithium at all, but these "lithium waters" were sought as a cure for rheumatism, diabetes, asthma, gout, and every other imaginable ailment. People also prized them for what were widely believed to be their general health-promoting properties and both bathed in and drank the waters.

Lithia Springs, Georgia, was among the most prominent of the U.S. spas. As far back as the fourteenth century, the Cherokee considered these waters to have sacred, healing properties. And for thousands of years this site was a spiritual, healing, and political center for the Cherokee tribes. By the late nineteenth century, the heyday of lithium water cures, Lithia Springs and its Sweet Water Hotel had become a major destination for the rich and famous. A train line ran directly from New York City to Lithia Springs. Presidents Cleveland, Taft, McKinley, and Theodore Roosevelt and Mark Twain and the Vanderbilts were among those who came to Georgia to "take the waters."

But the spas, although located throughout Europe and the United States, were not sufficient to meet the public's demand for lithium water. "Please send me a case of Lithia Water as soon as possible," President Cleveland wrote in 1895 after visiting Lithia Springs, Georgia.[3] He was not alone in his enthusiasm for lithium water, and indeed, bottled lithium water seemed to be the answer. In short order, innumerable brands of bottled lithium water came on the market, each promising extraordinary health benefits. The public devoured it. And not just water. Lithia Beer, which was presumably brewed with lithium water from a well in the basement of the brewery, was promoted based on its lithium content.

Toward the end of the nineteenth century, at the peak of the craze for lithium water, chemists began to analyze these waters. It became clear that if the waters contained any lithium at all, it was in minuscule amounts. Some of the bottled water came from mineral springs that actually contained lithium, some of the "lithium water" had no lithium whatsoever, and some came with lithium added by the manufacturer. With the passage of the U.S. Pure Food and Drug Act in 1906, which mandated among other things that product labels accurately state the ingredients, federal prosecutors went after lithium water and the claims that it contained sufficient amounts of lithium to heal an assortment of ills. In a 1910 case regarding one of the best-known lithia waters, the Supreme Court of the District of Columbia concluded: "For a person to obtain a therapeutic dose of lithium by drinking Buffalo Lithia Water he would have to drink from one hundred and fifty thousand to two hundred and twenty-five thousand gallons of water per day. It was further testified, without contradiction, that Potomac River water contains five times as much lithium per gallon as the water in controversy."[4] Typical of these prosecutions, Buffalo Lithia Water lost the case. It had to change its name to Buffalo Mineral Springs Water.

As "natural" lithium water and manufactured bottled lithium water became discredited because of their uncertain lithium content and benefits, lithium tablets came on the scene. They could be added to water and other drinks, creating a more substantial lithium dose. As just one example, the Sears, Roebuck Catalogue of 1908 included Schieffelin's Effervescent Lithia Tablets. It advertised them as a treatment for a variety of uric acid afflictions. According to the Catalogue, a dose of "one tablet dissolved in a glass of water makes a very agreeable, refreshing and beneficial effervescing draught."[5]

By the early decades of the twentieth century, the uric acid diathesis had lost favor with physicians and lithium its stature as a cure-all, but well into the 1930s the public continued to think that lithium provided health benefits. The still popular drink 7 Up began life in 1929 as a patent medicine product called Bib-Label Lithiated Lemon-Lime Soda. Lithium citrate was one of its seven main ingredients and a key selling point. Soon after launch, its inventor changed the name to 7 Up Lithiated Lemon Soda, and in 1936 he shortened the name to 7 Up. The lithium was not removed until 1950 (in 1948 the FDA banned lithium from beer and soda drinks). The rationale for the name is unclear. A likely explanation is that it's a reference to the seven original ingredients. Some have suggested, perhaps more fancifully, that the name 7 Up is an allusion to the atomic weight of lithium (6.94).

In 1948, not long after the uric acid diathesis had lost its grip on medical thinking and lithium treatment had been deemed useless, lithium resurfaced, this time as a salt substitute. Doctors were recommending—as they still do—that people with heart failure and high blood pressure reduce their intake of sodium. Because table salt (sodium chloride) is a major source of sodium, doctors advised low-salt diets. To make such diets more palatable, lithium chloride, which has a salty taste (not surprising, since it is chemically similar to table salt), came on the market as a salt substitute, often in the form of a solution. Patients gobbled it up; it tasted like table salt and it was cheap. They sprinkled it liberally on their food. In short order, reports of lithium toxicity turned up and several patients died as a result of it.

Since lithium first surfaced as a medical treatment, its toxic properties have been of concern. In doses not much higher than those given as a treatment, whether for gout or bipolar illness, lithium takes on the qualities of a poison. People taking too much of it can suffer dizziness, nausea, vomiting, tremors, drowsiness, and blurred vision. If lithium isn't stopped, these symptoms can progress to seizures, coma, and death. This toxic potential of lithium is why measurement of its blood levels is a necessary part of treatment.

Garrod had noted some of lithium's toxic effects, and throughout the late nineteenth and early twentieth centuries, sporadic reports about lithium toxicity appeared, but these were largely ignored. In contrast, the lithium toxicity that occurred in the wake of its use as a salt substitute got extensive publicity. Both the medical establishment and the general public reacted with alarm.

In 1949, the FDA ordered the manufacturers of salt substitutes to take them off the market. In retrospect, the salt substitute idea was not a happy one. People on low-sodium diets are particularly prone to lithium toxicity—they tend to retain lithium in the body—and, coupled with its unregulated consumption, this use of lithium chloride nearly led to a public health disaster. Although the salt substitute brouhaha came to a quick conclusion and was limited to the United States, it had far-reaching consequences. After Cade detected lithium's effectiveness in mania, both he and other Australian psychiatrists were at first slow to take it on because of worries about toxicity fueled, in part, by the salt substitute debacle. And lingering concerns about lithium's toxicity accounted to some extent for the 20 years it took after Cade's breakthrough before the FDA allowed doctors to prescribe lithium in the United States.

The salt substitute fiasco positioned lithium in both the public's mind and that of the medical profession as a potentially dangerous substance, best avoided. So John Cade's original 1949 report of lithium's benefit in mania could not have arrived at a less propitious time. But arrive it did, and in retrospect it is acknowledged as a revolutionary advance, one that ushered in the modern era of psychiatric treatment.

4

Breakthrough

WHEN HE returned from Changi in September 1945, Cade, like the other former POWs, was a walking skeleton. The formerly robust and athletic Cade weighed about 90 pounds. He recuperated for a short time at Heidelberg Hospital, near Melbourne, and then on January 1, 1946, he rejoined the Victoria Mental Hygiene Department, this time as director of the Bundoora Repatriation Mental Hospital.

Cade's original intent when he left the Department of Mental Hygiene to join the army was to open a private practice upon his return, as did many of his medical colleagues. But his time in Changi had left him brimming with research ideas, and public psychiatry gave him the opportunity to pursue them. Beyond the specific notions that he sought to test, Cade had come to believe that all psychiatrists should undertake some sort of research. In concluding a 1951 lecture about psychiatric research, Cade said: "Let each one of us engaged in the treatment of mental illness deliberately set out to investigate for ourselves some one of the numerous problems which arise, according to our own particular training or enthusiasm. Let us never rest content with the present bounds of knowledge."[1] Although Bundoora was small as Victorian mental hospitals went—it had just 200 patients—Cade felt that it provided ample opportunity for research. As he said to his wife Jean, when she asked him when he would pursue his original intent of opening a private practice, "I've decided not to . . . I can see many more patients here in a day than I'd ever see in private practice."[2]

The first idea that Cade decided to look into—one that had been brewing for a while—was the possibility that manic-depressive illness occurs because the body produces an unusual amount of a normal substance. Drawing an analogy between manic-depressive illness and thyroid disease, Cade reasoned that like thyrotoxicosis and myxedema (hypothyroidism), which come about when the thyroid gland produces too much and too little thyroid hormone, respectively, mania occurs when the body produces too much of some substance and depression when it produces too little. In support of this hypothesis, Cade pointed out that patients in the throes of mania behave in many ways as if they are intoxicated—restless, disinhibited, noisy, flamboyant. He saw a parallel with the toxic state produced by too much thyroid hormone.[3] In fact, some of the typical symptoms of thyrotoxicosis—irritability, hyperactivity, sleeplessness—overlap with those of mania.

It is likely that Cade's belief that manic-depressive illness had a biological basis and, for that matter, that other serious psychiatric illnesses like schizophrenia did as well, arose at least in part from his experiences at Changi. He had observed the adverse effects of malnutrition and vitamin deficiencies on the POWs' psychological state. He had also noted that autopsies conducted on POWs who had suffered psychiatric illness often revealed tumors and other brain abnormalities. Moreover, Cade believed that the psychological explanations then in vogue for these mental afflictions—stress, adverse early experiences, and psychoanalytic formulations—didn't hold water. Further supporting a medical or biological basis for manic-depressive illness was, as Cade put it, the "absolute failure" of any sort of psychotherapy to influence the course of the illness. Speculating about the "essential nature of manic-depressive illness," Cade didn't pull his punches: "Psychopathological explanations seemed to me to be singularly unconvincing, and completely useless when it came to treatment or prevention of attacks."[4]

Fortified with a guiding hypothesis, Cade started to look for the substance that causes manic-depressive illness. He had no idea what the substance might be, but he figured that it would be easiest to find when it was produced in excess—that is, in mania—and that if the body produced an excessive amount it would show up in the urine.

Accordingly, Cade began to collect early-morning urine samples from patients on the wards of Bundoora Hospital. Because these urine samples were passed after 12 to 14 hours without fluid intake, they were quite concentrated and most likely to show the presence of the presumed toxic substance. He collected samples from patients with mania, depression, and schizophrenia, as well as from some healthy people.

Then Cade proceeded to carry out what he described as a crude toxicity test. Because he had no idea what the toxic substance might be or what effect it might have on animals, he decided to "spread the net as wide as possible and use the crudest form of biological test."[5] And crude it was. He simply injected various amounts of urine into the abdominal cavities of guinea pigs and determined the quantity required to kill them.

Cade, his wife Jean, and their four sons lived in a house on the grounds of the mental hospital. Cade kept the jars of patients' urine on the top shelf of the family's refrigerator and he housed the guinea pigs in the back garden, where they were treated as family pets as well as experimental subjects. His "laboratory," wherein he prepared solutions, analyzed urine, and injected the guinea pigs, was an unused pantry on one of the wards of the mental hospital. It contained, as his son Jack remembers it, "a bench, sink, a few jars of chemicals, some simple lab instruments (pipettes etc.)."[6]

Cade soon discovered that while any urine in sufficient quantity would kill a guinea pig, some of the urine specimens from manic patients were particularly lethal. For example, the urine from some manic patients would kill guinea pigs in a dose as low as 0.25 milliliter per 30 grams of body weight, whereas the lethal dose of the most toxic "control" urine (urine from patients with other diagnoses and from healthy people) was at least 0.75 milliliter per 30 grams.

Cade noted that when a guinea pig injected with urine died, the mode of death was the same, regardless of the source of the urine. For the first 20 minutes or so after getting injected with urine, the guinea pig seemed perfectly fine. But then it started to tremble and lose its balance. Soon after, it started to twitch, the twitching progressed to full-blown convulsions, and finally the guinea pig became unconscious and died in a state of status epilepticus (nonstop convulsions).

Because the mode of death was the same regardless of the source of the urine, Cade reasoned that the same toxic agent was at work. In an attempt to identify this toxic agent, Cade embarked on a series of modest experiments that now have a mythic place in the history of psychiatry. These experiments did not follow an entirely logical or readily understood sequence, and Cade misinterpreted one of the critical results, but his effort to find the toxic substance led him, albeit via a circuitous and serendipitous route, to his groundbreaking discovery.

First, Cade examined the toxicity of the common constituents of urine: urea, uric acid, and creatinine. These are all breakdown products of protein metabolism found in normal urine. He injected high concentrations of each of these substances into guinea pigs and found that the creatinine and uric acid didn't harm them but that urea killed them in the same manner as urine. So urea seemed to be the lethal element. But Cade's further investigations showed that urine from manic patients did not contain more urea than other urines and, furthermore, that the concentration of urea in manics' urine was not high enough to account for their toxicity. So some other factor had to account for the unusual toxicity of manics' urine, something that enhanced the toxicity of urea. Cade set about finding what that other substance might be.

I've read Cade's description of his next steps, the steps that led to the discovery of lithium's ability to relieve mania, more than a hundred times, and in a seminar I teach about discoveries in psychiatry I've gone over those steps with hundreds of students. Nevertheless, the rationale behind some of those steps continues to baffle us all.

As Cade described it, he decided to study the possibility that one of the common constituents of urine—creatinine or uric acid—made the urea in manic urine more lethal.[7] So, first he added creatinine to urea. But he found, in fact, that the creatinine prevented convulsions and death. (This inspired Cade, ever curious, to take a short detour from his inquiry into manic-depressive illness to try creatinine as a treatment for epilepsy. Using guinea pigs as his subjects, he got some promising results. However, owing to the expense of creatinine, the difficulty Cade had obtaining it in sufficient quantity, and the scarcity of suitable patients, he was not able to get beyond this preliminary stage. Cade considered the results of his work with creatinine in epilepsy to be promising but inconclusive. As far as anyone knows, neither he nor anyone else pursued the matter further.[8])

Cade continued to pursue the question of why urine from manic patients was so much more toxic than that from other patients. Creatinine itself didn't seem to be the answer; urine from manic patients did not differ from other urines in creatinine content, and the possibility that some substance in urine from manic patients neutralized creatinine's protective action did not strike Cade as a likely explanation. What about uric acid? In a preliminary experiment, Cade had found that uric acid increased slightly the toxicity of urea. But uric acid did not seem a likely culprit. Cade postulated that even if the toxicity of urea were maximally enhanced by uric acid, the urine specimens from manic patients were still more toxic than could be explained by the concentration of urea. Cade wondered if those urine specimens contained a third substance that enhanced the toxicity of urea. But he was at a loss as to what this substance might be, and to his disappointment he never did discover it.

It's not completely clear why he decided next to further explore the impact of uric acid on the toxicity of urea. There are no apparent biochemical grounds for suspecting uric acid, and Cade's preliminary research suggested that uric acid had a minimal effect on urea's toxicity. But because this was a move that turned out to have far-reaching consequences, it would be nice to know what lay behind it. Unfortunately, Cade doesn't spell out his rationale for taking another look at uric acid; he merely says, "It now appeared important to estimate more accurately how much uric acid increased the toxicity of urea."[9]

I met with my next-door neighbor, a chemist involved in drug development research, to try to learn something about the basic chemistry behind Cade's lithium studies—the fate of lithium salts in solution, the molecular weights of the lithium compounds, elementary acid-base chemistry, that sort of thing. When I told him that I had difficulty making sense of Cade's shift to uric acid, he pointed out that I was seeking logic where it doesn't necessarily play much of a role. "I can completely understand it," he said. "The guy was stuck, he was looking around his lab, saw a bottle of uric acid on the shelf, and figured, 'I'll try adding some more of this.'"[10]

As his first foray into the more complete study of uric acid, Cade wanted to inject guinea pigs with a solution that contained both urea and a high concentration of uric acid. But he came up against the practical problem that uric acid does not readily dissolve in water. So, as a way of getting both urea and uric acid into guinea pigs, he made up a solution containing urea and the most soluble salt of uric acid—lithium urate—and injected that into guinea pigs. Unexpectedly, the lithium urate seemed to reduce the toxicity of urea. In further experiments, he found that another lithium salt, lithium carbonate, also protected guinea pigs from urea's toxicity. (When he injected guinea pigs with an 8 percent solution of urea, 5 out of 10 died; when lithium carbonate was added to the urea solution, all survived. This suggested that it was the lithium ion that conferred the protective effect.

Given the robust—and unexpected—results when Cade injected the solution containing urea and lithium salts, he decided to see if lithium salts by themselves "had any discernible effects on guinea pigs." Indeed they did. When he injected his guinea pigs with "large doses" of a 0.5 percent solution of lithium carbonate, he noted that "after a latent period of about two hours the animals, although fully conscious, became extremely lethargic and unresponsive to stimuli for one to two hours before once again becoming normally timid and active." Cade went on to say: "Those who have experimented with guinea pigs know to what degree a ready startle reaction is part of their make-up. It was thus even more startling to the experimenter to find that after the injection of a solution of lithium carbonate they could be turned on their backs and that, instead of their usual frantic righting reflex behavior, they merely lay there and gazed placidly back at him."[11]

Given lithium's apparent ability to tranquilize guinea pigs, Cade thought it would be worthwhile to try lithium salts as a treatment for mania, and he proceeded to do just that. Some believe that the readiness with which Cade went from these unexpected observations in guinea pigs to a treatment trial in manic patients defies scientific logic. More than a few who have examined and written about his discovery of lithium's effectiveness in mania believe that a good deal of serendipity was at play. Although Cade acknowledged that he made a bit of a conceptual leap, he maintained that his shift from sedated guinea pigs to manic patients was reasonable. In the 1949 paper where he first reported his landmark lithium discovery and in articles and lectures about the discovery over the next 30 years, Cade claimed that he had followed a logical sequence: "It may seem a long way from lethargy in guinea pigs to the control of manic excitement," he said, "but as these investigations had commenced in an attempt to demonstrate some possible excreted toxin in the urine of manic patients, the association of ideas is explicable."[12]

As the years went on, Cade dismissed with characteristic humor—and some irritation—the notion that serendipity or blind guesswork accounted for his discovery:

> People inevitably ask why lithium should have been tried in the treatment and prophylaxis of affective illness and especially, in the first place, of manic episodes. It is, of course, a perfectly valid question. Why not try potable pearl, or crocodile dung or unicorn horn? I was asked by a reporter some years ago—I thought rather unkindly—whether I had discovered it whilst shaving one morning.
>
> It is naturally the profoundest mystery unless one is aware of the preceding and intermediate steps. Then it can be seen, with such hindsight, to have been the almost inevitable result of experimental work I was engaged in, in an attempt to elucidate the aetiology of manic-depressive illness.[13]

Be that as it may, Cade's discovery that lithium had a profound influence on the behavior of guinea pigs is what prompted him to try lithium in patients, and that discovery was strictly serendipitous, an accidental by-product of his attempt to find the toxic element in urine.

Further, Cade's interpretation of lithium's effect on the guinea pigs, that it sedated or tranquilized them, an interpretation that suggested its potential benefit in mania, also points to the fact that something less—or more—than pure scientific logic was at play. For it now seems clear that the lethargy of Cade's animals was not a result of sedation but rather of lithium toxicity; in all likelihood, Cade's guinea pigs endured not a beneficial tranquilizing effect of lithium but rather early signs of lithium poisoning, which typically include lethargy and lack of responsiveness. Other investigators who later gave guinea pigs and other animals lithium were unable to reproduce the inactivity that Cade observed unless they injected the animals with large toxic doses.

Mogens Schou was a strong advocate of Cade and his lithium

work; he almost single-handedly took up the lithium mantle and did the research that firmly established its value. Schou offered this summary of Cade's guinea pig research: "The hypothesis which started his work was crude. His experimental design was not particularly clear. And his interpretation of the animal data may have been wrong. Those guinea pigs probably did not just show altered behavior; they were presumably quite ill. Nevertheless—and this is the marvel of the thing—a spark jumped in John Cade's questing mind, and he performed that therapeutic trial which eventually changed life for manic-depressive patients all over the world."[14]

But before Cade could undertake a therapeutic trial, he had to figure out what dose of lithium to use. This is not a trivial matter. We now know that the dose of lithium that works as a therapy is quite close to the dose that produces toxicity (nausea, vomiting, tremors and, if the lithium is not stopped, coma and death). If the dose Cade chose had been too low, the lithium would have been ineffective; if too high, the patients would have gotten ill. Either way the trial would have failed. As it turned out, Cade ended up prescribing lithium in doses that were near optimal and are in fact similar to the doses now in common use. Experts in pharmacology remain baffled by how Cade managed to come up with the right dose. Cade himself suggests that he just got lucky. In reminiscing about his discovery 20 years later, he said: "The original therapeutic dose decided on fortuitously proved to be the optimum, that is 1200 mg [milligrams] of the citrate thrice daily or 600 mg of the carbonate."[15] But given the effectiveness of the dose he decided on, some have speculated that along with Cade's good luck a bit of conscious deliberation may have been at play. So how did Cade arrive at a lithium dose that was so correct, a dose that allowed him to show lithium's value as a treatment?

The large doses he had given the guinea pigs did not offer adequate guidance on what dose would be safe and effective for humans. But recall that during the century before Cade's discovery, physicians had used lithium salts to treat gout and a wide array of other conditions, including some psychiatric ones, presumed to arise from excess uric acid. Both the medical literature and pharmacopeias of the late nineteenth and early twentieth centuries contained recommendations about suitable lithium doses for some of these disorders. Yet, as far as Cade—or probably anyone else—knew, lithium had never been given to manic patients, certainly not in the forms that Cade intended to use it (lithium carbonate and lithium citrate). So although Cade had access to information about what doses could be tolerated, he had no specific guidelines as to what dose would work.

The person before Cade who seems to have come closest to using lithium as a treatment for mania, and the first person on record to explicitly use lithium for that purpose, was William Hammond, Surgeon General of the United States Army during the Civil War and later a prominent neurologist and professor of diseases of the mind and nervous system at New York's Bellevue Hospital. As previously mentioned, in his 1871 textbook on diseases of the nervous system, Hammond reported that he had gotten good results when he used lithium bromide to treat acute mania: "Latterly I have used the bromide of lithium in cases of acute mania, and have more reason to be satisfied with it than any other medicine calculated to diminish the amount of blood in the cerebral vessels, and to calm any nervous excitement that may be present. The rapidity with which its effects are produced renders it specially applicable in such cases."[16]

Hammond prescribed high doses (up to 10 times the dose now used), which makes it hard to know if it was the antimanic effect of lithium, the sedative properties of bromine, or toxic reactions to one or both that produced the results.

Cade did not mention Hammond in his writings or lectures and in all likelihood he was unaware of Hammond's lithium therapy. In fact, Hammond's lithium work was largely unknown until the 1980s, when several lithium researchers learned of it and when Vibram Yeragani and Sam Gershon published a letter in the journal *Biological Psychiatry* in which they called attention to it.[17]

It is not surprising that Hammond's account of lithium as a

treatment for mania had stayed essentially unknown. It was buried in one paragraph of a 754-page textbook published 80 years before Cade launched the modern era of lithium treatment. And Hammond himself seemed to have abandoned lithium as a treatment for mania; he did not mention it in his later books. Some have speculated that he stopped recommending lithium bromide for mania because the high doses he had used produced lithium and or bromine toxicity.

So Cade didn't have much guidance from the medical literature about what dose of lithium to try in manic patients. As he pointed out in his landmark paper describing lithium as a treatment, he consulted a number of sources for information about lithium dosage. The esteemed *British Pharmacopoeia*, a leading source of drug information, gave the dose of lithium citrate as simply 5 to 10 grains and of lithium carbonate as 2 to 5 grains (the citrate and carbonate were the two recommended lithium preparations). But as Cade pointed out, these dose ranges were of little value for therapy, since they didn't specify how often the dose should be given. David Culbreth's *Manual of Materia Medica and Pharmacology*, another authoritative drugs reference, recommended, in 1927, higher doses—10 to 30 grains of lithium citrate and 5 to 15 grains of lithium carbonate. Cade also mentions that in 1859 Garrod, in his renowned (at the time) book about gout and related diseases, recommended treatment with lithium carbonate in doses of 1 to 5 grains, two to three times daily.

Cade was well aware from the medical experience with lithium over the previous 100 years that excessive consumption of lithium could produce an array of troublesome side effects, from upset stomach to "cardiac depression," but the available reference works did not offer information on the toxicity of the doses that Cade was thinking of using. He was concerned about the safety of lithium: "The older pharmacopoeias did not describe any toxic effects of lithium salts," he wrote, "but was that good enough?"[18] To address uncertainty about the safety of an untried treatment, there is always, as Cade put it, "the number one experimental animal, oneself." So with that in mind, and faithful to the medical principal *primum non nocere* (first, do no harm), Cade took lithium himself to see if it produced ill effects before giving it to patients.

Starting in early February 1948, he took single and repeated doses of lithium citrate and lithium carbonate and continued to do so for two weeks. Cade doesn't record what doses he consumed but recounts that they were the doses he contemplated giving to patients. His wife Jean, a nurse, was dismayed that Cade was experimenting on himself. According to Cade's son Jack, Jean was not happy about the jars of urine stored in the family refrigerator either, but she was even more distressed when Cade began consuming lithium. She recalled that after he started taking lithium, "I looked at him the next day, and the weeks that followed and wondered what I would do if he was changed by the lithium."[19] As it happened, Cade suffered no discernible ill effects, and on March 29, 1948, he started a manic patient on lithium for the first time.

This first patient, WB, had suffered symptoms of mania and depression for 30 years and had been confined to Bundoora Hospital for the past five years with unrelenting symptoms of mania. He was, as Cade put it, "a little wizened man of 51 who had been in a state of chronic manic excitement for five years . . . restless, dirty, destructive, mischievous and interfering. He had enjoyed preeminent nuisance value in a back ward for all those years . . . had long been regarded as the most troublesome patient in the ward . . . and bid fair to remain there for the rest of his life."[20]

In telling the story of his lithium discovery years later, Cade provided slightly more detail about WB's treatment than he did in his original 1949 report or in his case notes and records. Here's what he had to say in 1977, much of which follows his original report verbatim:

He [WB] commenced treatment with lithium citrate 1200 mg thrice daily on 29 March, 1948. On the fourth day, the optimistic therapist thought he saw some change for the better but acknowledged that it could have been his expectant imagination (it was April Fool's Day!). The nursing staff were non-committal but loyal. However, by the fifth day it was clear that he was in fact more settled, tidier, less disinhibited and less distractible. From then on there was steady improvement so that in three weeks he was enjoying the unaccustomed and quite unexpected amenities of a convalescent ward. As he had been ill so long and confined to a closed chronic ward he found normal surroundings and liberty of movement strange at first. Owing to this, as well as housing difficulties and the necessity of determining a satisfactory maintenance dose, he was kept under observation for a further two months.

He remained perfectly well and left hospital on 9 July 1948, on indefinite leave, with instructions to take a maintenance dose of lithium carbonate, 300 mg twice daily. The carbonate had been substituted for the citrate as he had become intolerant of the latter, complaining of severe nausea. He was soon back working happily at his old job.

It was with a sense of the most abject disappointment that I readmitted him to hospital six months later as manic as ever but took some consolation from his brother who informed me that Bill had become overconfident about having been well for so many months, had become lackadaisical about taking his medication and had finally ceased taking it about six weeks before. Since then he had become steadily more irritable and erratic. His lithium carbonate was at once recommenced and in two weeks he had again returned to normal. A month later he was recorded as completely well and ready to return to home and work.[21]

Over the ensuing 11 months, Cade went on to treat nine more manic patients with lithium and saw equally good results. Remarkably good, actually. He also gave lithium to six patients who had dementia praecox (now known as schizophrenia) and three who were chronically depressed.

Cade treated the patients with both lithium citrate and lithium carbonate, the lithium salts recommended in the pharmacopoeias and used in the nineteenth century to treat uric acid conditions. Cade started off using the citrate because it is more soluble and apparently better absorbed than the carbonate. But he found that patients tolerated the carbonate better, had less stomach upset, and he began relying on the carbonate preparation. After treating this first group of manic patients, he began using the carbonate exclusively, in 300 mg tablets, and that's how lithium is given today.

Cade wrote detailed notes about the patients on one side of lined cards. He also noted the patients' progress in their medical records but did not provide as much detail regarding lithium treatment and response as on the cards. These cards are now in the Medical History Museum of the University of Melbourne.

Cade generally started the patients on 20 grains of lithium citrate three times daily. On this dose their manic symptoms subsided within a week or so, and several weeks after that Cade started to reduce the dose. A few patients developed symptoms of lithium toxicity, primarily stomach discomfort, which Cade dealt with, quite correctly it turns out, by temporarily stopping the lithium and resuming it at a lower dose or substituting the carbonate for the citrate. Most of these original patients continued to take lithium for months or years at doses ranging from 10 grains of lithium citrate daily to 5 grains of lithium carbonate twice daily.

A grain is an old unit of weight, around since antiquity, originally based on the weight of a single grain of wheat or barley. Drug doses were commonly designated in grains until in the twentieth century the metric system gradually replaced the assorted older measurement schemes. Today, prescriptions rarely designate the dose of a drug in grains, but the grain is still used to measure the weight of bullets, gunpowder, and arrows. A grain is exactly 64.799 milligrams (mg) and is commonly approximated as 60 or 65 mg.

In his original report of the lithium study, Cade indicated the lithium dose in grains, but as the years went on he referred to those doses in the more contemporary milligrams. As had been customary in using lithium salts as therapy in the previous century, the dose of lithium citrate that Cade applied was twice that of lithium carbonate. (The lithium ion makes up a far smaller proportion of lithium citrate than it does of lithium carbonate; the amount of lithium in lithium citrate is only 40 percent the amount of lithium in a similar weight of the carbonate. Cade assumed (correctly), on the basis of his guinea pig experiments, that the lithium ion itself was the agent producing the clinical effect. Thus, he made sure that in using the two lithium salts, he was dispensing roughly equivalent doses of lithium, and to achieve equivalent doses required roughly twice the dose of lithium citrate.)

As Cade pointed out, the lithium dose he began with, indicated in his original report as 20 grains of lithium citrate three times daily (which in retrospect he referred to as "1200 mg of the citrate thrice daily or 600 mg of the carbonate"), turned out to be the "optimum." In fact, it is well within the therapeutic dose range applied in contemporary practice.

Cade did not spell out the process he went through to arrive at the lithium dose. He tells us only: "As lithium salts had been in use in medical practice since the middle of the nineteenth century, albeit in a haphazard way with negligible therapeutic results, there seemed no ethical contraindication to using them in mania, especially as single and repeated doses of lithium citrate and lithium carbonate in the doses contemplated produced no discernible ill effects on the investigator himself."[22]

Although Cade could not have known in advance which lithium dose would alleviate manic symptoms, and so he was indeed lucky to come up with a starting dose that was effective, it seems likely that his choice of dose rested on some thoughtful deliberation. We can't know what Cade was thinking, but it seems clear that the doses he took himself, and later gave to patients, were informed by the guidelines for lithium use in gout and other conditions provided in the pharmacology books he referred to in his original report. For example, Culbreth's 1927 *Manual of Materia Medica and Pharmacology*—cited by Cade—specified the dose of lithium carbonate as 5 to 15 grains and of lithium citrate as 10 to 30 grains. Although this and other pharmacology reference works did not say how often the dose should be repeated each day, one could presume, as Cade put it, "the traditional two to three times." Thus, it is noteworthy, and may not be coincidental, that the dose Cade settled on—20 grains three times daily—was right in the middle of Culbreth's recommendation.

Cade's report of the lithium trial in manic patients appeared in the September 3, 1949, issue of the *Medical Journal of Australia*.[23] It became that journal's most frequently cited paper, and even now, almost 70 years after its publication, remains one of that journal's most highly cited. Cade began the paper with a brief discussion of lithium's medical use in the nineteenth century and some of its side effects. He then touched on his lithium experiments in guinea pigs. He described the animals' apathy after he injected them with lithium carbonate and then explained that "in view of their sedative effect . . . it appeared worthwhile . . . to try lithium salts in the treatment of . . . mania."

Cade went on to provide brief vignettes of the 10 manic patients he treated with lithium. Three of the patients had chronic mania (a rare condition) with unrelenting manic symptoms for two to five years, and the remaining seven patients had the more typical recurrent episodes of mania, the most recent lasting several weeks to several months. As was the case with WB (the first patient), all of these patients showed unprecedented, dramatic improvement within a week or two of getting lithium. By the time he wrote the paper, presumably soon after March 4, 1949 (the last date mentioned in the case vignettes), five patients had improved sufficiently to leave the hospital, two of whom had been persistently manic for five years.

According to the published vignettes, four patients experienced side effects related to lithium toxicity. In three, the side effects resolved within a few days of stopping lithium, and the lithium was successfully resumed at a lower dose or with substitution of lithium carbonate. One patient, TF, who had endured chronic mania for over two years, recovered within two weeks of starting lithium but had persistent stomach trouble despite a reduction in lithium dose and switch to the carbonate. Cade stopped the lithium treatment. Two weeks later the patient had "drifted back to his previous manic state." Cade noted that two other patients, including WB, who had stopped lithium treatment for six weeks or more, had a return of manic symptoms only to have them quickly recede when the lithium was resumed.

All the published case vignettes, with the exception of TF's, ended with the patient continuing to take lithium and no longer manic. But not everything that happened to these patients made it into Cade's paper. After he submitted his paper for publication, he continued to record his observations about the patients on the lined cards and in their medical records. Several patients whose vignettes in the published report ended with them doing well had a somewhat less happy outcome as time went on.

WM's published vignette ended in late February 1949, after he had been on lithium for two weeks. Previously "garrulous, euphoric, restless and unkempt," he was now "practically normal—quiet, tidy, rational, with insight into his previous condition." According to the case notes, he continued to show "tremendous improvement," no longer requiring sedation and isolation, through early March 1949. But on April 10, 1949, Cade noted "anorexia, unsteadiness, general malaise and depression." On that date Cade stopped the lithium.

WS's published vignette ended on March 4, 1949. At that point he had been on lithium for several weeks and was well on the road to recovery. WS's improvement, like that of the other patients, was unprecedented. "An acquaintance who has known the patient for years," Cade wrote, "reports that he has never seen him as normal as at present." But WS did not continue entirely in this vein. In the case notes of March 10, 1949, six days after the published description, Cade wrote that WS had "slipped a bit" and was "rather garrulous." Accordingly, Cade increased his lithium dose. On March 15, WS was still garrulous and now complaining of diarrhea. At that point, Cade stopped the lithium.

WB, Cade's first patient, who had responded so dramatically both to treatment with lithium and to its removal, had a rocky time of it over the next two years. He remained outside the hospital for months at a time and worked intermittently, but he did not take lithium regularly and vacillated between periods of mania, when he was off lithium, and stomach upset when he was on it. In March 1950, noting that WB still had "dyspepsia, anorexia and vomiting," Cade stopped his lithium. "Under all circumstances," Cade wrote, "it seems that he would be better off as a free restless case of mania rather than the dyspeptic, frail little man he looks on adequate lithium." Two weeks later, Cade notes, "he was rapidly reverting to his manic phase and forgetting his dyspepsia."[24]

One month later, in the face of WB's unrelenting mania, Cade seemed to change his mind. In his note of May 3, 1950, he wrote that WB "has continued manic, restless, euphoric, noisy, dirty, mischievous, destructive, flight of ideas and thoroughly pleased with himself. His state seems as much a menace to life as any possible toxic effects of lithium. Therefore recommence lithium citrate gr. 20 tds. today."[25]

Within two weeks, WB was "quieter but miserable and asthenic." Cade discontinued the lithium, but WB started to go downhill. Over the next few days he became semicomatose and had three seizures. WB died on May 23, 1950. Cade recorded as the primary cause of death "toxaemia due to lithium salts, therapeutically administered."[26] He also listed inanition (exhaustion from lack of nourishment) and chronic mania among the causes of death. No autopsy was performed. The coroner's inquest, required by law when someone died while a patient in a mental hospital, included a deposition by John Cade. The coroner accepted Cade's conclusions regarding the reasons for WB's demise.

Had the eventual outcomes of these three patients been included in Cade's paper, lithium's side effects and toxicity would have figured in it more prominently, and lithium would have appeared a bit less promising. WB's death occurred eight months after the paper appeared, so it could not have been included. We don't know the exact date that Cade submitted his paper to the *Medical Journal of Australia*, but it's fair to presume that it was somewhere between March 4, 1949, the last date recorded in the published vignettes, and September 3, 1949, the date of publication. (Cade does not note the date he sent his paper to the journal, and the *Medical Journal of Australia* doesn't have editorial records from that era.) Because Cade wrote the notes about WS's and WM's side effects, and the fact that he stopped their lithium, on March 15, 1949, and April 10, 1949, respectively, it is not unreasonable to assume that he sent his paper off before he knew of these end results.

Whether or not Cade could have (or should have) included these two instances of lithium toxicity in his published paper has no bearing on the fundamental importance and validity of his discovery (both patients improved with lithium). There is no indication that Cade deliberately omitted this information from his published report; none of the dozens of psychiatrists and historians who have written about and scrutinized Cade's lithium research have suggested that he purposely excluded any data, and he did not avoid the problem of lithium toxicity in general. He discussed it at some length in his paper, detailed its symptoms, emphasized its dangers, stressed the importance of watching patients closely for its emergence, and provided guidance on how to manage it. Nonetheless, in light of the fact that in discussing his research over the years Cade seemed, at times, to overlook a number of pertinent matters, these possible omissions warrant some attention.

More problematic—and inexplicable—than the fact that two of Cade's patients did not eventually do as well on lithium as his report suggests is that time and again Cade described WB as a case of successful lithium treatment without ever mentioning that he eventually died from lithium toxicity. When in the 1960s lithium started to be widely studied and used, Cade was lauded for his discovery, and he was called upon to recount the "story" of his breakthrough at conferences, in journal articles, and in books. In his half-dozen or so published accounts of the "story," Cade described his guinea pig research and then went into a description of WB's pathway through lithium treatment, describing him as the "very first manic patient ever deliberately and successfully treated with lithium salts." The description regularly concludes with WB restarting lithium after undergoing a relapse and "completely well and ready to return to home and work."[27] WB is the only patient that Cade portrays in these accounts; as a result, WB has achieved a sort of prominence as a poster child for lithium, or at least Cade's poster child.

It is difficult to dismiss Cade's failure to mention WB's demise as a simple oversight. With one exception, Cade's contemporaries, as well as the psychiatrists and historians who have scrutinized his lithium research, have not taken him to task over this omission. The exception is Johan Schioldann, a Danish psychiatrist who emigrated to Australia and published a book in 2009 (*History of the Introduction of Lithium into Medicine and Psychiatry*) that challenges both Cade's status as the man who introduced lithium into psychiatry (Schioldann thinks that honor belongs to Carl and Fritz Lange) and Cade's account of his research. "It can be argued," Schioldann wrote, that it was "strongly misleading when Cade characterized WB as a 'successful' case of lithium therapy."[28]

Neil Johnson, a British psychologist who has written and edited several books about lithium, admired John Cade as a scientist and person, and in the context of Johnson's interest in lithium the two men became friends. In his well-known book *The History of Lithium Therapy*, Johnson says: "There is evidence that Cade was deeply troubled by the toxic side effects of lithium, to an extent which did not communicate itself in print."[29] Indeed, Cade's worry about toxicity prompted him to stop studying and using lithium soon after he completed his clinical trial and to discourage others from using it as well.

Schioldann suggests that Cade's silence about WB's death is evidence of his failure to communicate his concerns in print. We will never know if Cade's silence on this matter was a deliberate attempt to conceal a painful truth or in part or whole an unintentional lapse. Whatever the case, in omitting WB's fatal lithium toxicity from the retrospective versions of his lithium discovery, Cade painted a mistakenly rosy picture of this first patient's experience with lithium. WB's happy outcome became an integral part of the lithium story.

In May 1970, for example, an article appeared in *The Australian Women's Weekly* about Cade and lithium. It was titled "New Key to Mental Health," and it was based on an interview with Cade shortly before he left for the United States to receive an award for his lithium discovery. The article includes a few paragraphs about the first patient to get lithium, WB. After hearing about how much he improved on lithium, we learn that "on a maintenance dose of the drug each day, the patient remained normal for the rest of his life."[30]

While WB's death from lithium toxicity has no relevance to the significance of Cade's discovery, his consistent failure to mention it may well point to the sort of things that motivated him and how he coped with unpleasant realities. WB's death was not the only matter of some importance that Cade may have overlooked. Schioldann marshals a book's worth of evidence, albeit all indirect, suggesting that Cade knew of the Lange brothers' previous work with lithium, work that clearly suggested its potential value in the treatment of recurrent depression—not the same thing as mania or manic-depressive illness, but in the ballpark—and chose to disregard it.

To be sure, the sort of "evidence" that Schioldann puts forward is less than entirely convincing. He contends that Cade would almost certainly have known about the uric acid diathesis concept because it was so widely believed, even if in the previous century; and about the rationale it provided for the treatment of psychiatric symptoms with lithium; and in particular about the Langes' use of lithium in depressed patients. Although Carl Lange's original report of his seminal studies on periodic depression appeared in Danish, Kraepelin referred to this work in the eighth (1913) edition of his classic psychiatry text (in German); and an English translation of Kraepelin's chapters on manic-depressive illness came out in 1921. Schioldann alleges that Cade would have known of Lange's work from this English edition, "which without much doubt . . . he would have studied from cover to cover."[31]

Unquestionably, Cade was familiar with Kraepelin's views on manic-depressive illness; he discussed them in his own 1979 book about psychiatry, and as an honors medical student and a well-read and knowledgeable psychiatrist, he almost certainly read Kraepelin early in his career. But whether Cade came across and attended to Kraepelin's brief—and dismissive—mention of Lange's work is anyone's guess.

Cade has also been mildly criticized for another "oversight"; in his retrospective accounts of his lithium discovery and the further development of lithium, he recognized the key role of Mogens Schou in confirming and extending the therapeutic use of lithium, but he did not mention other researchers who made significant contributions. Some feel that his disregard of Edward Trautner's decisive work with lithium levels, which, as we shall see, went a long way toward rescuing lithium treatment from obscurity, is particularly perplexing.

Explanations for Cade's oversights or selective forgetting run the gamut. One account suggests that Cade's failure to mention WB's demise from toxicity arose from his profound embarrassment over this event. This theory, posited by a contemporary of Cade's, points out that Cade's father (also a psychiatrist) wanted him to become Australia's greatest psychiatrist. It might have been very important to Cade not to disappoint his father, making WB's death especially mortifying.

Barry Blackwell, a British psychiatrist who moved to the United States and who for a while was volubly skeptical about the value of lithium and skeptical as well of Cade's seemingly unassailable saintlike status, attributed Cade's oversights to cryptomnesia, a kind of selective forgetting often motivated by an unconscious desire to embellish one's reputation and career by claiming the contributions of others as one's own.[32] Blackwell also raised (less plausibly) the possibility that Cade's "forgetting" to mention Trautner, Sam Gershon, and some other lithium pioneers in a 1970 talk about the lithium discovery was a sign of early dementia. Cade was 58 at the time and there is no indication that he suffered from dementia then or later.[33]

But as pertinent as Cade's memory "lapses" may be to an understanding of who he was and to an accurate view of his character, equally pertinent is the almost total absence of criticism directed to him or his methods. Schioldann and Blackwell are among the very few who have raised any questions about Cade's behavior and methods. The vast majority who have written and spoken about Cade and his research, many of whom are fellow Australians, simply lavish him and his scientific approach with praise. They don't mention Cade's selective forgetting or his methodological foibles. Schou's positive spin on Cade's somewhat inexplicable move from intoxicated guinea pigs to manic patients reflects a common view: "To make therapeutic discoveries on the basis of misinterpreted experiments requires curiosity, daring, luck, and compassion for the patients."[34] Even Schioldann, Cade's foremost critic and the only one who has taken him on in print, edges up to questioning his ethics and methods but stops short of explicitly accusing him of deliberately withholding information, using flawed methods, or providing a misleading account of his research.

One reason for the reticence to criticize Cade comes from the fact that any hint that his conduct was less than exemplary is hard to square with the prevailing view of him as a man and scientist of impeccable integrity. "An honourable, upright Christian gentleman, honest in all his dealings, and with a vast fund of kindly human feeling and consideration" seems to have been the almost universal assessment.[35]

Also deterring criticism is Cade's well-deserved status as a war hero. It seems both unjust and mean-spirited to disparage someone who endured the horrors of Changi and did so much to protect his men and keep up their morale. Several years ago, I was discussing with a prominent Australian psychiatrist Schioldann's implied disapproval of Cade for his failure to mention earlier psychiatric work with lithium. It is in fact an egregious breach of research ethics to disregard the related prior contributions of others, and my Australian colleague, who has written several articles about Cade and his research, was well aware of this and of the ambiguities around Cade's apparent neglect of previous lithium work. But with tears in his eyes he said, "There's no way I'm going to criticize that guy. After what he went through at Changi he's a war hero and I'm not about to say anything bad about him."

Whether or not Cade deserves censure for overlooking the efforts of others and whether he discovered or, as Schioldann would have it, "rediscovered" lithium as a psychiatric treatment does not bear on the significance of his breakthrough. Cade's 1949 paper, and not any of the related work that preceded it, clearly showed that lithium alleviates mania, described how it could be applied in the treatment of patients, and was sufficiently compelling to prompt others to do the definitive studies that established lithium's usefulness. Even before it was verified and extended by Schou and others, Cade's research in 1948 and 1949 revolutionized the treatment of manic-depressive illness and the outlook for its victims. Cade is rightly credited for launching the "psychopharmacological revolution," for showing that a drug can relieve mental symptoms.

Cade also showed in this one small study that the beneficial effect of lithium salts come from the lithium ion itself, not from a specific salt of lithium or the acid fraction of the salt. And almost as important as Cade's demonstration that lithium relieves mania was his finding that lithium's benefit is highly specific. Whereas three of the six patients with dementia praecox (schizophrenia) whom Cade treated with lithium "lost their excitement and restlessness and became quiet and amenable for the first time in years," Cade noted that none of these patients showed improvement in the fundamental symptoms typical of the disorder; their delusions and hallucinations continued unabated.[36]

Because lithium reduced the symptoms of mania, Cade wondered if it might bring on an episode of depression. He saw no evidence of this in the 10 patients he treated for mania, and when he gave lithium to three patients with chronic depression, he found that the depression neither improved nor worsened. Cade concluded: "The effect on patients with pure psychotic excitement—that is, true manic attacks—is so specific that it inevitably leads to speculation as to the possible aetiological significance of a deficiency in the body of lithium ions in the genesis of this disorder."[37]

Now, almost 70 years after Cade wrote this, lithium's specificity as a primary treatment for manic-depressive illness exclusively continues to give it a unique position among psychiatric drugs. The other drugs used in psychiatry—the antidepressants, antipsychotics, and antianxiety agents—relieve a wide array of symptoms and are effective, more or less, in an assortment of conditions.

Cade's speculation that lithium's specificity might shed light on the basis of manic-depressive illness was also prescient. Although a simple "deficiency in the body of lithium ions" does not appear to account for this disorder, lithium's singular effectiveness continues to guide research efforts. When scientists finally elucidate the way that lithium alleviates and prevents episodes of manic-depressive illness, we will be far closer to understanding the roots of this problem.

When Cade's patients with mania began getting better, he knew he was onto something. In the year or so before his report came out, he gave talks at hospitals and gatherings of psychiatrists throughout Victoria describing the remarkable therapeutic effects of lithium. Soon after his paper appeared, though, reports of death from lithium toxicity started to appear, and Cade became wary of lithium and stopped using it. Still, over the next two decades, lithium started to be widely studied and regularly and safely used. By the late 1960s, it was clear that lithium offered unprecedented benefits to people with manic-depressive illness. The psychiatric community acknowledged Cade as the discoverer of lithium treatment, and the accolades started pouring in. By all accounts, Cade reveled in his renown and was enormously gratified by the reception, albeit late in coming, that he and lithium received.

Although Cade basked in his fame and was not shy about describing his research with lithium, his view of how he came up with his discovery—and in particular how much deliberation as opposed to luck was at play—seemed to vacillate. On the one hand, he strenuously objected to the idea that serendipity played a part. He insisted that since his guinea pig experiments were an attempt to illuminate the cause of manic-depressive illness, his jump to testing lithium in manic patients was part of a logical sequence. All the same, he suggested on more than one occasion that he came upon lithium as a result of some lucky puttering about. In reminiscing about his lithium discovery, he once said: "I am not a scientist. I am only an old prospector who happened to pick up a nugget."[38] And along similar lines, Cade was notably—and publicly—self-effacing about his scientific and research credentials. From a 1951 address on psychiatric research: "My qualifications for discussing medical research in general or even psychiatric research in particular are best left unstated. I might most kindly describe myself as an enthusiastic amateur, full of curiosity, with fair determination, golden opportunities, inadequate knowledge and woeful technique. But even the small boy, fishing after school in a muddy pond with string and bent pin, occasionally hauls forth a handsome fish."[39]

Cade's colleagues seemed to agree with his self-assessment. "If anyone was fated to stumble across the anti-manic properties of as unlikely a substance as lithium," wrote Neil Johnson, "it was surely John Cade: he was probably less of an 'investigator,' in the strict sense, than an 'enquirer,' turning over the stones of the scientific environment to see what interesting things might be wriggling about underneath."[40]

Indeed, Cade came to his lithium studies with little research experience and no formal research training. Nonetheless, he was far from naive about research methodology and how to interpret results. He was in fact a thoroughly well-informed psychiatrist, familiar with research developments and knowledgeable about the requirements of a treatment study. Here's what he said about methodological issues in his 1949 paper:

> In the treatment of such a self-limiting disorder as mania, the therapeutic innovator must be more than ordinarily on his guard. Whether this or that treatment is of any value must be carefully assessed from as many angles as possible. With an episodic disorder of this type, the efficacy of a particular treatment may be judged by one or more of the following criteria. The more criteria that are satisfied, the more sure are we that it is a treatment of real and not suppositious value.
>
> 1. Improvement must proceed pari passu [side by side] with treatment.
> 2. Chronic cases are of special value in assessment because in them spontaneous remission is far less likely to occur in a specified short period than in the recent cases.
> 3. Supporting evidence may be forthcoming from the treatment of non-manic psychotic excitement.
> 4. The ideal is, of course, the method of controlled observation of a sufficient number of treated and untreated patients. The disadvantage of the ideal is that mania is not so common a psychotic disorder as might be thought and it would take any one observer even in a large mental hospital probably some years to accumulate a large enough series to be statistically significant. But although the first three criteria may be insufficient for formal proof, they are capable of giving strong circumstantial evidence for or against efficacy.[41]

Cade believed that his results were unequivocal. "There is no doubt," he wrote in concluding his paper, "that in mania patients' improvement has closely paralleled treatment and that this criterion has been fulfilled in the chronic and subacute cases just as closely as in the cases of more recent onset. The quietening effect on restless non-manic psychotics is additional strong evidence of the efficacy of lithium salts." And so this small study, which would probably not be published today and which lacked the standardized assessment methods, statistical niceties, and other accoutrements of contemporary research, yielded results that changed the practice of psychiatry and mended the lives of millions.

Cade was 37 years old when his 1949 paper appeared. He never did any further research with lithium. As the years went on and psychiatrists worldwide were prescribing lithium, Cade wrote a few articles and book chapters reviewing what was known about lithium treatment and recounting how he discovered its antimanic properties. But it was, as we shall see, left to others to take up the mantle and do the research that firmly established lithium's value.

The last survivor of the original 10 manic patients died of natural causes in 1980 at the age of 76. He had been on lithium for more than 30 years. John Cade died the same year.

5

Aftermath

WHEN A new treatment comes along that promises to heal an intractable condition, physicians—and the public—are usually quick to embrace it. In a typical scenario, after a brief period of caution and skepticism, doctors begin to use the treatment with increasing frequency and confidence. At first they prescribe it just for the illness in which the originators showed it to be effective; but if the treatment proves useful, it doesn't take long for medical professionals to try it—often rather indiscriminately—for a wide array of other disorders. For a short time, some of these disorders, in the eyes of the beholder at least, seem to improve. (The nineteenth-century medical dictum "Use new drugs quickly while they still work" has lost none of its relevance.) Eventually, as more information accrues, reality tempers unbridled enthusiasm and doctors eventually prescribe the treatment selectively, where it has true benefit. New treatments of today follow this path, much as they did in Cade's time.

Lithium did not follow the standard route of a new drug. It took a full 20 years before psychiatrists accepted and routinely prescribed lithium, and the FDA did not authorize its use until 1970. By contrast, psychiatrists rapidly and enthusiastically took on the psychotropic drugs introduced just a few years after lithium—antipsychotics and antidepressants—and within a year or two, regulatory agencies approved them.

Why the slow acceptance of lithium? First, since lithium is a natural substance, drug companies could not patent it, so it was of no commercial interest and no drug company promoted it. Second, drug companies vigorously marketed the psychiatric drugs that came on the scene soon after lithium, and the psychiatric community seized upon these new agents. Moreover, the new drugs turned out to offer some benefit (but not as much as lithium) to people with manic-depressive illness. These drugs became the rage, and in doing so drew attention away from lithium. Further, as Cade himself pointed out, the fact that his discovery "was made by an unknown psychiatrist, working alone in a small chronic hospital with no research training, primitive techniques and negligible equipment was hardly likely to be compellingly persuasive, especially in the United States."[1]

Notwithstanding all of the above, the major impediment to lithium's acceptance was its potential toxicity. That lithium could have unpleasant and dangerous effects was well known. Reports of its toxicity in both animals and people had appeared sporadically during the 100 years before Cade's work. But although lithium's dangers had been well documented, they had not been a cause for concern. Doctors had stopped prescribing lithium as a treatment in the late nineteenth century, and the lithium water, so avidly consumed in the late nineteenth and early twentieth centuries, contained negligible amounts of lithium, not enough to pose a hazard. All this changed at the beginning of 1949. At that point, just eight months before Cade published his lithium paper, a panic erupted over lithium's toxicity in connection with another use for it.

As discussed in chapter 3, lithium's troubles began in 1948

when several U.S. manufacturers came out with lithium chloride as a salt substitute for people on low-salt diets. Lithium chloride does indeed taste salty, and grateful patients, instructed to eliminate ordinary table salt from their diets because of heart or kidney disease, readily welcomed this stand-in. It usually came as a solution—a concoction called Westsal was a popular one—and customers, liberated from an unpalatably bland diet, gobbled the stuff up. Unlike the lithium water so fashionable in the previous century, the salt substitute solutions contained large concentrations of lithium (Westsal was 25 percent lithium chloride).

Given what was already known about lithium's toxicity and the readiness with which it appears when people consume large amounts of lithium, what happened next should not have come as a surprise: some of the people using the salt substitute became gravely ill—weakness, nausea, tremors, and blurred vision, progressing in some instances to unconsciousness and death. Lithium soon emerged as the culprit, and it became clear that sodium depletion as a result of a low-salt diet increased the susceptibility to lithium poisoning. People on low-salt diets were, in fact, the last people who should have been imbibing lithium; with a reduction in salt (sodium) intake, the body retains more lithium, setting the stage for lithium poisoning. In addition, the blandness of low-salt diets prompted some folks to ingest huge amounts of the lithium salt substitute.

In February 1949, a number of doctors sent reports describing patients with lithium toxicity to the *Journal of the American Medical Association* (*JAMA*). Four reports depicted a total of 14 patients with lithium poisoning, 3 of whom had died. They came out in the March 12, 1949, issue of *JAMA*, but even before they appeared, Morris Fishbein, editor of the journal, asked newspapers and radio stations to issue warnings about lithium's dangers.[2] In mid-February, American newspapers and radio broadcasts started to carry stories, based largely on the accounts sent to *JAMA*, about people becoming ill and dying as a result of the lithium chloride salt substitute. Over the next few weeks, newspapers throughout the country carried stories of several additional deaths and more than a few episodes of serious illness ascribed to the lithium salt ("Salt Substitute Kills 4" ran a headline in the *New York Times*).[3] There seemed to be a burgeoning epidemic of lithium toxicity. The AMA and FDA put out warnings about the hazards of the lithium salt substitutes, and they didn't pull their punches. An AMA spokesman described the salt substitute as a "slow-acting poison," and the FDA warned people who had purchased lithium salt to "stop using this dangerous substance at once." On February 18, the FDA ordered lithium salt manufacturers to take their products off the market. Health officials from New York to Los Angeles immediately banned their sale. In New York City, 40 health inspectors canvassed wholesale and retail druggists, searching for and confiscating bottles of lithium salt.

By March, the lithium toxicity panic had subsided, leaving in its wake a handful of lawsuits and the widespread belief that lithium is dangerous stuff. The lithium salt substitutes had had a short and geographically limited life span, and the outbreak of lithium toxicity that they produced was confined to the United States. Nonetheless, as fleeting as the panic about lithium was, it was also profound, reverberating beyond U.S. shores and influencing attitudes about lithium, particularly in the United States but elsewhere as well, over the ensuing decades. Cade does not mention the salt substitute debacle in his 1949 lithium paper, but by the time his paper appeared, word of it had reached Australia.

The July 30, 1949, issue of the *Medical Journal of Australia* included a note entitled "Salt Substitutes and Lithium Poisoning." It covered the four *JAMA* reports in some detail and ended with a warning: "Lithium chloride appears to present an important problem. It seems reasonable to suggest not only that physicians should exercise care and constant supervision when it is in use, but that they may well think twice before prescribing it at all." This warning was just as applicable to any lithium containing salt, including the lithium carbonate and lithium citrate that Cade had prescribed for his manic patients.

It's not clear when Cade learned of the salt substitute poisonings, but at the time he wrote his lithium paper he was clearly aware of lithium's potential to cause harm. In his report, he issued a cautionary note about the symptoms of lithium "over-dosage"—stomach pain, nausea, vomiting, tremor, slurred speech, and muscle twitching. "Unless such symptoms are followed by immediate cessation of intake," he wrote, "there is little doubt that they can progress to a fatal issue." He warned that patients should be watched carefully for symptoms of overdose.

Cade continued to be concerned about the damage that lithium could do. Soon after his lithium paper appeared, the October–December 1949 issue of the Australasian Association of Psychiatrists' quarterly newsletter carried the following note:

LITHIUM TREATMENT OF MANIA. (Ref. M.J.A., September 3, 1949, p. 349): Dr. Cade wishes to collate all evidence relating to the above form of therapy, which has established a degree of success, but is still to be regarded as being in the experimental stage. He wishes to be able to obtain a broader view of—(1) its therapeutic results, and (2) its toxicity. He especially stresses the importance of careful clinical observation when maximum doses are being employed and the need for prompt withdrawal when toxic symptoms appear. He would desire communications to be addressed to him—Dr. John F. J. Cade, Repatriation Hospital, Bundoora, Victoria.

Meanwhile, in the year or so before his original paper came out in print, Cade had read it and talked about the results to gatherings of psychiatrists throughout Victoria. So by the time his paper appeared, about a half-dozen Australian psychiatrists, most working in long-term mental hospitals, had started giving lithium to patients with manic-depressive illness and some other conditions as well.

It wasn't long before Australian psychiatrists began to publish reports about their experiences with lithium, one of them a cautionary tale. The first published account following Cade's paper turned up a year later in the August 12, 1950, issue of the *Medical Journal of Australia*. It had the less-than-encouraging title "A Case of Chronic Mania Treated with Lithium Citrate and Terminating Fatally." Edgar Roberts, a psychiatrist at Ballarat Mental Hospital, a large asylum 65 miles west of Melbourne housing about 1,000 patients, described what happened when he gave lithium to two patients—one "constantly maniacal," the other schizophrenic. Roberts had followed Cade's treatment protocol to the letter, giving each patient 20 grains of lithium citrate three times daily. Both patients became quieter after one week of treatment, but the patient with mania showed signs of lithium toxicity. Despite discontinuation of lithium, she began to have seizures and then slipped into a deep coma. Nine days after the onset of toxic symptoms she died. Roberts concluded that "as a form of symptomatic treatment lithium citrate suffers from the grave disadvantage that the therapeutic dose is dangerously close to the lethal dose."

Three weeks later, Dr. J. V. (Val) Ashburner, a psychiatrist at Sunbury Mental Hospital on the outskirts of Melbourne, came out with a brief letter in the September 2, 1950, issue of the *Medical Journal of Australia*, responding to Roberts's concerns. Ashburner had attended a meeting where Cade read his forthcoming lithium paper, and soon after, inspired by Cade's results, he had started treating patients suffering various forms of excitement with lithium salts, primarily lithium carbonate (which the hospital pharmacist had on hand). Ashburner gives few details in his letter, but does point out that he treated more than 50 patients, that about a dozen were able to leave the hospital, and that patients with mania were more likely to improve than those whose excitement arose from other causes.

Ashburner's observations regarding lithium's safety were as significant as his findings about lithium's value. "Minor toxic manifestations are not uncommon," he said, "but I have never yet seen any toxic symptoms which failed to clear up within twenty-four to forty-eight hours after the patient stopped taking the drug."

Ashburner's work did not constitute a formal research study (for that matter, neither did Cade's). He simply wanted to learn more about what sounded like a promising treatment. Still, his letter is the first published confirmation of Cade's lithium results. "It is already possible to state, unequivocally," Ashburner wrote, "that the cases treated at this hospital amply confirm the value of Cade's discovery, . . . an important original contribution to the treatment of psychiatric patients." He concluded, "It would be a pity if Dr. Roberts's communication were to create an unfavorable impression."

But Roberts's report of a lithium fatality and talk in the Australian psychiatric community of several other lithium-related deaths, alongside the U.S. salt substitute disaster, did indeed create an unfavorable impression, not least on John Cade himself. The reported instances of lithium-induced illness and death, combined with his own encounters with lithium toxicity, convinced Cade that lithium's potential for harm outweighed its benefit, and he stopped using it. He also discouraged its use among his colleagues, more than a few of whom had been captivated by lithium's promise.

When, in 1952, Cade became superintendent of Melbourne's prestigious Royal Park Mental Hospital, he banned the use of lithium at that institution. Cade remained at Royal Park until his retirement in 1977. As its superintendent and dean of its Clinical School, he stood among Australia's prominent psychiatrists, and his prohibition of lithium hindered, albeit for a short while, both research on lithium and its use as a treatment. Sam Gershon, today an eminent psychopharmacologist and one of the founders of lithium treatment, recalls that as a young psychiatrist he became aware of Cade's lithium research and, having landed at Royal Park in 1952 for a year of psychiatric training, hoped to work with lithium. He was dismayed to find that by the time he arrived, Cade had outlawed lithium. Eager to find out more about this promising new treatment, Gershon left Royal Park after nine months to pursue studies of lithium at Ballarat and other mental hospitals.

So, by the end of 1950, although lithium had been given to psychiatric patients throughout Australia, lithium treatment for mania was essentially unknown elsewhere; and, given persistent concerns about its toxicity and Cade's opposition to its use, lithium was teetering on the brink of oblivion. As it turned out, two researchers, one working in Buffalo, New York, and the other in Melbourne, saved lithium from the dustbin of medical obscurity.

John H. Talbott was a professor of medicine at the University of Buffalo's medical school when in 1948 he was asked to examine one of the lithium chloride salt substitutes. Although he did not provide the brand name of the salt, given its composition it was probably Westsal. He carried out his studies in 1948 and 1949, concluding them after the salt substitute panic and publishing the study report in January 1950.

Talbott was an expert both in gout and in human metabolism, particularly in the way the body adjusts to shifts in salts and other chemicals. He had a long-standing interest in identifying a salt substitute for people on low-salt diets. Along with his expertise in biochemistry, Talbott had a penchant for casting a skeptical eye on simplistic explanations and for challenging medical beliefs not grounded in actual data. His know-how and his willingness to challenge prevailing wisdom served him well in his investigation of the lithium chloride salt. He was methodical and thorough; and although his studies were not intended to inform lithium's use as a psychiatric medicine, they made it possible for lithium to undergo further development as a treatment.

Talbott started off by supplying the lithium salt solution to more than 50 hospital patients who, because of heart or liver disease, were on low-salt (sodium chloride) diets. He instructed them to use as much lithium salt as necessary to make their food palatable. The patients ended up consuming an average of 500 mg per day. Only three patients developed symptoms similar to those in the reports of toxicity. The symptoms were mild and, as Talbott pointed out, might well have been caused by the the patients' medical treatments or underlying diseases.[4]

To see if larger amounts of the lithium salt had ill effects, Talbott gave six patients and four healthy people 2 to 5 grams of lithium chloride daily, up to 10 times the amount required to make food palatable. The only symptom encountered was stomach upset. It cleared immediately after stopping the salt intake.

He gave rats the human equivalent of 7.5 grams per day of lithium chloride, 15 times the amount required to make food adequately salty. The rats showed no signs of toxicity, and autopsies revealed no damage to their organs or cells.

Talbott followed over 50 patients who regularly used the lithium salt on their food for more than three months and tracked more than a dozen such patients for longer than six months. He encountered no instances of either mild or severe toxicity. With few exceptions, patients liked using the lithium salt; they found that it gave their food an agreeably salty taste. Ever the thorough researcher, Talbott, his son recalls, brought some of the lithium salt home and asked his family to judge its saltiness.[5] On the basis of his observations, including the enthusiasm of the patients who used it on their food, Talbott concluded that lithium chloride was a suitable salt substitute and should be made generally available.

But Talbott didn't stop there. He started to investigate the relationship between the amount of lithium ingested, the serum level of lithium, and symptoms of lithium poisoning. He gave both healthy people and hospital patients large doses of lithium carbonate (the equivalent of four to nine times the amount of lithium salt used to flavor food) and observed both their symptoms and serum concentrations of lithium. Some of the people who got these high lithium doses suffered lithium side effects or toxicity, including stomach upset, drowsiness, and tremors. Talbott found that the presence of these symptoms correlated with the serum lithium concentration. No symptoms cropped up when the serum level of lithium was below 0.7 millequivalent (mEq) per liter. Further, Talbott stated that with one exception he did not see clear signs of lithium intoxication until the serum level reached 2.3 mEq per liter.

Talbott continued his studies through the lithium toxicity scare and did not complete them until after lithium salt substitutes had been taken off the market. In concluding his report, he scrutinized the accounts of supposed lithium poisoning that had started the lithium panic. He pointed out that several of the victims had taken enormous amounts of lithium salt (up to eight times the average amount used by Talbott's patients) and that both the symptoms and the deaths attributed to lithium might well have been the result of the severe diseases suffered by these people, including heart failure and diabetes, and might have also come from their low-salt diets. "It was impossible to ascribe the reported deaths to the ingestion of lithium," Talbott wrote, "since there were other complicating factors, each of which could have been responsible for the death of critically ill persons."[6]

Talbott, a feisty, wiry 5 feet 7 inches, who, as one of his colleagues put it, "appeared much larger when angry,"[7] did nothing to hide his displeasure over the media's role in the lithium scare. In the article reporting the results of his lithium studies, he wrote:

Near the conclusion of these studies, I was notified that a death alleged to be associated with excessive lithium intake had been reported to the manufacturers. I also learned that after a conference with the Federal Food and Drug Administration all lithium substitutes for salt had been withdrawn from the market and steps had been taken to recall outstanding stocks. One manufacturer immediately mailed a letter to all physicians notifying them of this step and of the reported possibility of untoward effects. Ten days after the withdrawal from the market the report of several deaths, alleged to have been caused by lithium poisoning, was broadcast. No advance notice of this broadcast, in order that physicians could prepare the several thousands of patients taking these salt substitutes for the alarming statements, was given the physicians, druggists or manufacturers by those responsible for the dissemination of the report. The prescribing physician was embarrassed in many instances by a deluge of telephone calls from his patients requesting advice, and the only information available was that reported over the air and in the newspapers. It is believed that the situation was not so serious as one was led to believe from the lay reports."[8]

Talbott did his best to counter the irrationality behind the lithium scare. "The incidence of valid reactions due to the ingestion of lithium is unknown," he said. "Following the indiscriminate press and radio publicity an attempt was made in this clinic and others to contact hundreds of lithium users in order to obtain more precise information. The alarm had so frightened the majority of those who used the substitute that many symptoms, regardless of cause, were attributed to the ingestion of lithium. I myself have seen several patients claiming lithium intoxication whose symptoms, on close inquiry, were found to be due to other causes."[9]

Talbott's work made a strong case for the value and safety of the lithium salt substitutes. But it came too late to stem the flood of alarm; once banned, the salt substitutes remained off-limits and have not been heard of since. Nonetheless, Talbott's demonstration that lithium toxicity was related to serum lithium levels—that if the serum lithium level was measured such toxicity could be avoided—laid the groundwork for lithium to be developed as a treatment.

Talbott went on to become a prominent American physician. He edited the prestigious *Journal of the American Medical Association* and the *Merck Manual*, the world's most widely used medical text. But his role in the development of lithium treatment, critical as it was, remained largely unknown, even to himself. After his salt substitute studies, he did no further research with lithium, and although he lived until 1990, well after lithium had been established as a major psychiatric treatment, it seems that he never knew of the crucial part he played in making lithium a viable treatment. Talbott had a long career as a physician, researcher, and medical writer and editor. He dedicated himself to alleviating the suffer-

ing caused by gout and arthritis and studied the body's response
to extreme environmental conditions—for example, frostbite in
extreme cold and heart and lung adaptations in high altitude. But
he did not tackle mental illness. As it turns out, however, his work
with lithium was not his only unintended contribution to psychiatry. Talbott's son, John A. Talbott, is today an eminent psychiatrist
and former president of the American Psychiatric Association.

In concluding his report on the lithium salt substitutes, Talbott
wrote: "Untoward reactions following the use of lithium were
not found . . . except in association with serum lithium concentrations above 1.0 milliequivalents." Talbott was spot-on. Today,
patients taking lithium have their serum lithium level measured on
a regular basis. The designated safe upper limit is 1.2 mEq, almost
exactly where Talbott put it.

Talbott's contribution to the progress of lithium was an unintended consequence of the thoroughness with which he examined
lithium salts. But at the same time, on the other side of the world,
a scientist named Edward Trautner, working in the Department of
Physiology at the University of Melbourne, was quite deliberately
setting out to confirm and extend Cade's observations regarding
lithium's astounding benefit in mania—and to figure out a way to
work around its toxicity so that it could be applied as a treatment.
Trautner had read Talbott's report. Guided by it, he resolved to
measure serum lithium levels in a study examining lithium's therapeutic and toxic effects in psychiatric patients. That study was the
first to measure lithium levels in conjunction with lithium's use
as a medicine and, along with the ones that Trautner and his colleagues did next, made it possible for lithium to come into its own.

Eduard (later known as Edward) Trautner arrived in Australia
in early September 1940 as a German refugee. He was one of the
2,542 so-called enemy aliens deported to Australia by the British
government in July 1940 on the *Dunera*, a ship that achieved notoriety for the appalling conditions of its voyage to Sydney. (Meant
to hold 1,600, the ship was badly overcrowded. Men had to sleep
on the floor and on benches, only 10 toilets were available, sewage

flooded the decks, and the British guards confiscated and looted luggage and frequently beat the passengers.) Most of the people deported were Jewish refugees and others who opposed the Nazi regime and had fled Germany. At the outbreak of war, fearing that in the event of an invasion men of German and Austrian origin living in Britain would aid the enemy, the British government, without distinguishing among those who did and did not actually represent a security risk, rounded up these foreign nationals, temporarily interned them, and then proceeded to deport them.

Trautner—Trautie to his colleagues and friends—had been born in Berlin, where he spent the first half of his life. He served in the German Army during the First World War and after the war got his medical degree and practiced medicine. Trautner was a maverick on several fronts. He was born into a Catholic family, but according to Sam Gershon, his student, research collaborator, and friend, he was a "devout atheist." Trautner was also a socialist and vocal anti-fascist. In trouble with the Nazi Party, he fled Germany in 1933, just before the Nazis came to power. According to some accounts, he ended up in Spain during the Spanish Civil War and from there went to Britain. At some point along the way, he studied several sciences, including botany and biochemistry. Forcibly deported from Britain on the *Dunera*, he landed in Sydney only to be sent to an internment camp in Tatura, central Victoria.

R. Douglas Wright, a professor of physiology at the University of Melbourne, found out that Trautner was interned in Tatura and in 1942 arranged for him to join Melbourne's physiology department. Trautner worked there for the next few years, developing procedures for extracting pharmaceutical products from plants. After the war, Trautner went back to England for a brief stint at Oxford's School of Botany and then returned to join Wright in Melbourne, this time to carry out investigations on nervous tissue metabolism.

Trautner was a scientific polymath—his expertise ranged from animal and plant physiology to brain biochemistry—and he had his fingers in all sorts of research pies. Charles Noack, a new psychi-

atrist on the staff of Melbourne's Mont Park Hospital and Trautner's former student, had heard of Cade's lithium work and was
interested in examining what seemed like a promising treatment.
Noack turned to Trautner for help in planning and implementing a
lithium investigation. Trautner seems to have immediately grasped
the significance of Cade's observations and the importance of lithium toxicity. He and Noack proceeded to carry out a study that
now stands beside Cade's as one of the founding stones of lithium
treatment.

Noack and Trautner gave lithium citrate and carbonate to over
100 psychiatric patients, more than 30 of whom had mania. With
lithium's toxicity and the recent lithium fatalities in Australia well
in mind, Trautner had a particular interest in looking at the relationship between lithium's beneficial effects and its toxic symptoms. Noack and Trautner started out with the same lithium doses
used by Cade. They carefully watched patients for signs of lithium
toxicity, and they reduced the dose or temporarily stopped the
lithium entirely if symptoms of toxicity occurred. Mindful of Talbott's findings on the relationship between lithium poisoning and
serum levels, they decided, along with meticulous observation of
patients' symptoms, to measure their serum levels of lithium.

Theirs was the first attempt to measure serum lithium levels
during lithium treatment of mania (now these levels are routinely
measured), and they were able to pull this off because of Victor
Wynn, a young Research Fellow in the Physiology Department.
Wynn is another one of those folks who, like Talbott, made an
unwitting but vital contribution to lithium's progress.

As a medical officer in the Australian Army, Wynn had seen
some soldiers with kidney failure and dangerously high blood levels of potassium. After the war, he wanted to pursue research on
potassium and more generally on fluid and electrolyte balance.
With that in mind, he joined the Physiology Department at the
University of Melbourne as an unpaid Research Fellow.

The body's electrolytes—chemical substances like potassium,
sodium, and calcium—have to be maintained in a fairly narrow

range for cells and tissues to work properly. Methods for measuring them, whether for clinical or research purposes, should be accurate and practical. The available techniques were cumbersome, inaccurate, and time-consuming, so Wynn personally raised the money to buy a flame spectrophotometer, a new device recently introduced by the Beckman Instrument Company, which made it possible to measure electrolytes speedily and with high precision. Wynn then set up a laboratory within the Department of Physiology centered around this technology. His research group set about investigating, among other things, electrolyte and water balance in both sheep and humans.

The flame spectrophotometer, which Wynn and his group were using to quantify sodium and potassium in biological fluids, could also be used to measure lithium, a similar chemical. Trautner asked Wynn if he would run some serum samples through his flame spectrophotometer to assess lithium levels, and Wynn readily agreed. A postgraduate student working in Wynn's lab recalls Trautner's cheery persistence: "Trautie assured Charlie Noack . . . that it would be no trouble to me to run a few lithium samples through for him. I forget how many thousand samples I finally did during the period."[10]

Noack and Trautner reported their results in the August 18, 1951, issue of the *Medical Journal of Australia*.[11] Their study established several key points, all of which have withstood the test of time. First, lithium, just as Cade had said, alleviated symptoms of mania. All but one of their more than 30 manic patients improved, and many continued on lithium and remained well during more than a year of observation. Noack and Trautner also observed that lithium was beneficial in preventing recurrences of mania and, consistent with Cade's observation, that it had little impact on depression or the fundamental symptoms of schizophrenia.

As noteworthy as lithium's benefits, lithium was safe. None of the more than 100 patients treated with lithium died or developed serious toxicity. Some showed signs of lithium "intoxication"— stomach upset, dizziness, tremor—but these abated with dose adjustment. Nonetheless, Noack and Trautner acknowledged that lithium was not "invariably safe." They called attention to the three recent lithium-related fatalities in Australia—the patient reported by Roberts and two others. In view of the fact that these patients suffered convulsions followed by coma, symptoms not seen in other instances of lithium poisoning and death, they speculated that these patients had an unusual predisposition to "lithium-caused collapse."

Finally, Noack and Trautner showed that serum lithium levels could be practically monitored. The levels they observed were consistent with Talbott's; the average was about 1.0 mEq per liter and the highest level they saw was 2.1 mEq per liter in a patient with no signs of poisoning.

Noack and Trautner concluded that "we did not meet with any serious cases of intoxication among over 100 patients suffering from different mental diseases. In view of the very beneficial effect of the drug in the cases of mania reported, it does not appear to be justified to abandon lithium as a form of medication solely because some fatal cases have been reported in which lithium poisoning has been incriminated."[12]

Noack and Trautner's work has been overshadowed by Cade's and mostly overlooked. Yet experts in psychopharmacology who have scrutinized lithium's progress agree that, as the lithium historian Neil Johnson put it, their paper "was probably as influential as Cade's original report in promoting lithium therapy."[13] Summing up this phase in lithium's development, Ulrich Schäfer, another lithium scholar, declared: "Talbott, Noack and Trautner laid the foundations for further developments in the practical management of lithium treatment."[14]

Victor Wynn went on to a distinguished career as a professor of human metabolism at St. Mary's Hospital Medical School in London. The flame spectrophotometer was not his only entrepreneurial venture. In London he raised the money for and founded several research units and medical charities.

Charles Noack collaborated with Trautner on one more lithium study and after that did no further research.

Edward Trautner continued to do lithium research. He and his colleagues studied the effect of lithium on body chemistry and identified the specific serum levels of lithium required to achieve a beneficial effect, as well as those associated with toxicity and death. The levels they identified continue to guide lithium treatment. Gershon, who had remained interested in lithium, sought Trautner's guidance and joined him in these studies as a collaborator. Following his work with Trautner, Gershon left Australia and was instrumental in bringing lithium to the United States. Trautner left the Department of Physiology in 1961 and headed for the warmer climate of Queensland. He died in 1979 at age 93.

Among the consequences of Noack and Trautner's paper—and not the least of them—was that it got the attention of the Danish psychiatrist Mogens Schou. Upon reading it, Schou decided that further study was warranted, and he proceeded to do the first controlled study of lithium in mania. Over the next 50 years, Schou, at times single-handedly, carried out and nurtured lithium research. More than anyone, with the possible exception of Cade, he was responsible for establishing lithium as a major psychiatric treatment.

There was nothing accidental about Schou's lifelong connection to lithium. His father, Hans Jacob Schou, was a prominent Danish psychiatrist and, reminiscent of John Cade's father, was the director of two psychiatric hospitals, one for patients with epilepsy and psychosis and the other for patients with neuroses and "mild depressions." The elder Schou had a particular interest in manic-depressive illness. The pull of this ailment was not strictly academic. It was, as his son Mogens put it, "presumably not unconnected to the occurrence of manic-depressive illness in the family."[15] In fact, manic-depressive illness appeared in Mogens's younger brother, who suffered from severe recurrent depressions beginning at about age 20. Hans Schou believed that moods and disorders of mood, like manic-depressive illness, had a biological basis. Along with caring for patients—his primary work—he set up a research laboratory to study chemical and physiological changes in psychiatric disorders. He and his colleagues wrote scholarly articles about these matters and about the course and treatment of recurrent depression and manic-depressive illness.

Born in Copenhagen in 1918, Mogens Schou came of age at a time when there were no effective treatments for manic-depressive illness. Patients got rest cures, baths, and supportive psychotherapy, barbiturates for mania and opium for depression—all of little use. He had vivid memories of "depressed patients wandering in the hospital park with bent heads and anguished faces, waiting and waiting for the depression to lift and fearing manic and depressive recurrences." Schou remembered his father's exhilaration when in 1938 electroconvulsive therapy came out. Here was something that worked; within a matter of weeks, both depressions and manias could be brought to an end.

Inspired, he believes, by his father's example, Schou decided to study medicine with "a specific view to do research on manic-depressive illness." After getting his medical degree in 1944, he spent four years studying clinical psychiatry at several hospitals in Scandinavia. Frustrated by how little one could do to bring relief to psychiatric patients, Schou decided to specialize in biological psychiatry research. With the encouragement of Erik Strömgren, professor of psychiatry at Denmark's Aarhus University and an internationally esteemed psychiatrist, Schou spent two years doing basic biochemical research in the laboratories of two well-known biochemists (Herman Kalckar in Copenhagen and Heinrich Waelsch in New York). Schou returned to Denmark with skills in experimental biology under his belt, and with the support of Strömgren, then head of the Psychiatric Hospital in Risskov, Denmark, he started a research laboratory.

In 1951, soon after arriving at the Risskov Psychiatric Hospital, Schou was looking for a suitable research topic when Strömgren called his attention to Noack and Trautner's recently published article on mania and lithium. In short order, Schou got hold of Cade's paper. He was intrigued by the apparently striking benefits of lithium, and foreshadowing his lifelong quest to gain recognition for lithium, he wrote in his first paper on lithium that he found it "astonishing" that these Australian reports had not aroused greater interest among psychiatrists. Schou figured that part of the reason for the lack of interest was the toxicity problem; according to the Australian accounts, the doses required for a beneficial effect were close to those that produce toxic symptoms. Schou also thought that the studies to date might not have been fully convincing; the methods used had not eliminated common sources of error that can result in a treatment seeming to be effective when it isn't. These include the influence of suggestibility or wishful thinking on the part of both patient and observer and the fact that symptoms of mania come and go spontaneously, so when an improvement occurs during treatment it's hard to know if it's a result of the treatment or a spontaneous change.

Schou wanted to investigate the lithium treatment of mania in a way that would reduce the sources of error and thus provide more definitive proof of its effectiveness. With this in mind, he decided to conduct a double-blind, randomized controlled trial (RCT). The RCT is now the gold standard for treatment research; since the late twentieth century, it is the method most widely used, indeed required, to assess and confirm the value of new treatments. But in the early 1950s, when Schou did his lithium study, the RCT was a fairly new approach that had only recently been applied in medical research. (The first published RCT, a study of streptomycin in tuberculosis, came out in 1948.) Prior to this time, new treatments were assessed, if they were assessed at all, more or less the way Cade had evaluated lithium. A doctor tried a new remedy—a drug or surgical procedure—on a group of patients, and on the basis of how patients fared decided whether or not it was worthwhile. On the surface, this seems a not unreasonable approach. But over the first half of the twentieth century, researchers and statisticians from an array of fields—agriculture to psychology—came to realize that this sort of clinical impression, or seat-of-the-pants approach, to evaluation was apt to provide misleading results.

Schou and his colleagues confirmed the value of lithium in treating mania by carrying out one of the first, if not in fact the very first, RCT in psychiatry. The result, which verified lithium's unique healing properties, was a turning point for lithium and psychiatry. In view of the RCT's critical role in the development of lithium, it seems pertinent to look in some detail at the features of an RCT and what they are meant to accomplish.

The "controlled" feature of an RCT refers to what is probably the most critical part of the trial: the treatment under study is compared with a "control" treatment, often a placebo but sometimes an alternate treatment. The purpose of the control treatment is to abolish or "control for" the influence of so-called nonspecific elements on the outcome of the trial. These nonspecific elements include the features present in almost any treatment situation or healing environment: a medical evaluation; a chance to discuss one's condition; a diagnosis; a plausible treatment; the enthusiasm, commitment, and respect of doctors and nurses; the symbols and rituals of healing, including the doctor's office, stethoscope, and so forth; and, most important of all, the belief that improvement is in the offing. These common treatment factors can have a powerful impact on how people feel; they account in large part for the ubiquitous placebo effect. Over the history of medicine, these ingredients of treatment and the placebo effect they generate have accounted for the benefit, and are often the only benefit, of most apparent treatments.

By the time Schou was starting his lithium research, the medical research community had recognized that researchers needed to take into account such nonspecific treatment elements when evaluating how patients responded to a specific treatment, like lithium. They did this by comparing the experimental treatment—lithium, for example—with a "control" treatment, which would encompass the same nonspecific elements (a caring doctor, the same medical equipment in the office, and, most important, a plausible treatment). The control "treatment" was often a placebo. Once they were able to compare the two treatments, researchers could also confidently discount the influence of spontaneous changes in symptoms—changes like a sudden onset of euphoria or despair—that had nothing to do with the actual specific treatment. Such changes are a common feature of manic-depressive illness.

Randomization is the method by which subjects or patients in an RCT are assigned to one of the treatments under study. The point here is that the investigator does not decide which patients get an experimental treatment and which a control substance. Rather, a random process, essentially like a coin toss, determines who gets what. Randomization avoids so-called selection bias. If investigators allotted patients to treatment, it is likely that they would choose patients with certain characteristics to receive a particular treatment. Randomization ensures that the patients in each treatment group are comparable, allowing a fair test of the treatments.

And finally, whenever possible, blinding is incorporated into an RCT. When researchers know whether the patient is getting medicine or placebo, that knowledge invariably affects—largely unconsciously—how the researchers perceive the patient's progress. If, for example, the researchers know that the patient is on lithium (and they believe that lithium is valuable), they will be inclined to see improvement. And when patients know what treatment they are getting, that knowledge can sway—again, mostly unconsciously—how they feel and how they report their symptoms. The ideal is the "double blind," in which neither the patient nor the investigator knows what the patient is getting. In some circumstances, for practical reasons, the best that one can do is the single blind, where only the patient is blind (unaware of) the treatment.

The lithium experiment that Schou and his colleagues carried out was by today's standards rather haphazard, and given the importance of the question at hand, their methods were astonishingly simple; they used none of the embellishments—comprehensive, standardized evaluation procedures and complex statistics—that are part and parcel of today's treatment research. Nonetheless, their study included all the essential features of a modern RCT, and as subsequent research showed, the results were valid.

They treated 38 patients with mania, some of whom had prolonged manic episodes and others frequent short episodes. Some of the patients got continuous lithium on an open basis (both the patients and investigators knew that the patients were on lithium), and others underwent double-blind shifts between lithium and placebo about every two weeks. Schou designed the study, assigned the patients to lithium or placebo, measured serum lithium levels, analyzed the data, and wrote the final paper. He did not see or evaluate the patients. His collaborators—Strömgren and two other senior psychiatrists—treated and assessed the patients. Neither they, nor the ward staff, nor the patients knew whether the patients were taking lithium or placebo.

Schou sat in his laboratory and flipped a coin to decide who got lithium and who placebo. (Today researchers use a computer-generated table of random numbers to allocate patients to treatment, but Schou's coin flip achieved the same aim.) "I wouldn't say the nurses were entirely happy with the knowledge that some of their violent manic patients might be given placebo," he recalled years later. "Some of them even broke the tablets and tasted them. However, we had foreseen that and by adding various constituents to the placebo tablets made them similar to the lithium tablets in taste, color and consistency. So we fooled the nurses."[16] As a further safeguard of the double-blind, before patients swallowed them, the tablets were pulverized and mixed with a good quantity of sugar to mask any possible differences in taste.

Every day, the collaborating psychiatrists and ward staff rated the patients' mood and activity level on a three-point scale: +, ++, +++. On the basis of these ratings and chart notes, Schou classified each patient's response to lithium treatment as definite improvement (manic episodes stopped or manic symptoms decreased with lithium but not placebo); possible improvement (mania lessened during lithium treatment, but spontaneous improvement could not be excluded); and no improvement. Fourteen patients showed definite improvement, 18 possible improvement, and 6 no improvement. All got lithium, and some got a placebo as well. The paper reporting their research appeared in 1954.[17] Schou and his colleagues concluded, "Our results are in essential agreement with those of the Australian psychiatrists: lithium has an unquestionably beneficial effect on a number of manic patients." The placebo-controlled and double-blind elements of their trial allowed them to go one step further, and it was a crucial step. In "at least one-third of the cases," they wrote, "the clinical improvement observed during lithium treatment is not due to inaccuracies in clinical assessment, suggestibility or spontaneous variations."

Alert to the lithium toxicity issue, Schou and his collaborators noted that several patients in their study treated with relatively high doses of lithium (48 mEq per day, 1,800 mg per day) developed "slight toxic symptoms"—most frequently vomiting, diarrhea, and hand tremors. These symptoms did not occur at lower doses and disappeared in a few days when the lithium was stopped or the dose reduced. Schou and his collaborators also noted that the lithium dose required for a therapeutic effect was close to that which produced these side effects. One of the lithium-treated patients died of a stroke, which they considered unrelated to her treatment with lithium.

Despite the fact that their patients did not experience serious untoward effects from lithium, Schou struck a cautious note that typified his combination of scientific rigor and concern for the welfare of patients: "The fact cannot be excluded that lithium therapy may be dangerous under special conditions of which our knowledge is still insufficient. A careful clinical and biochemical control of patients under lithium treatment appears advisable for the time being."[18]

Following Noack and Trautner's lead, Schou measured serum lithium levels. Like Noack and Trautner, he found that they usually ranged from 0.5 to 2.0 mEq per liter, and consistent with Noack and Trautner's observations in their first study, Schou did not see a strong correlation between serum lithium and signs of toxicity. "Nevertheless," he wrote (presciently it turns out), "it is our impression that a knowledge of the serum lithium concentration is of some value as a guide for the therapy, and we should be hesitant to institute lithium therapy under conditions where the serum lithium level could not be checked regularly."[19]

The report of this study, 10 pages in all, is rich in detail and packed with gems that foretold a good bit of what later research and clinical experience revealed about lithium. For example, in this first study, Schou and his colleagues found that in some patients with frequent episodes of mania, lithium stopped the episodes. But at that point, Schou and his colleagues did not distinguish between the treatment of a manic episode and the prevention of such episodes. "We took it for granted that if a therapeutically active drug were given continuously, it must also prevent further recurrences."[20] Within a decade, lithium's unique prophylactic effect on both manic and depressive episodes was recognized, and this preventive feature has remained lithium's chief benefit.

Schou noticed that the effect of lithium was not simple sedation. Many of the patients who improved with lithium had been treated with massive doses of barbiturates and other sedatives without benefit; during treatment with lithium, patients did not appear "drugged" as they did with sedatives. The ensuing experience with lithium fully confirmed this observation.

Schou also recorded that some of the patients on long-term lithium treatment "did not feel quite their own self," or, as one put it, felt "kept down" by the medicine. Echoing that "kept down" feeling, some of today's patients complain that lithium blunts their feelings, perceptions, and creativity.

Among other things, Schou and his colleagues compared lithium with electroconvulsive therapy (ECT), then the only effective treatment for mania. They pointed out that while ECT can alleviate a manic episode, its effects are short-lived. Lithium, on the other hand, seemed to keep people in a normal state for as long as they took it. Right again.

Small, untidy, and rudimentary as it was, this study put lithium's unique benefit as a treatment for mania on solid ground. Yet more than a decade passed before the psychiatric community took much notice. Foretelling Schou's long struggle to gain recognition for lithium, the paper reporting this study, now considered groundbreaking by any standard, did not have an easy time getting into print. Schou sent it first to the prestigious and widely read *Journal of Mental Science* (now the *British Journal of Psychiatry*). Eliot Slater, an assistant editor at the journal—and eminent British psychiatrist—assessed the paper and turned it down, recalled Schou: "He did not think much of this report about an unknown drug and suggested that we send the manuscript to a more out-of-the-way journal, the *Journal of Neurology, Neurosurgery and Psychiatry*."[21] That journal did publish the paper, but it was indeed "out-of-the-way"; few psychiatrists read it, and the response to Schou's study was a rather deafening silence.

By the mid-1950s, lithium was languishing in the wake of the new psychiatric drugs. Still, Schou was convinced that he was onto something. From his first foray into lithium treatment, he recognized both its value as a therapy and its potential to shed light on the biological basis of manic-depressive illness. He considered doing basic laboratory studies to uncover the way lithium works—how it affects the brain—but since his laboratory in Risskov "could not compete with neurochemical institutes elsewhere with their surplus of expensive equipment, basic research on lithium's mode of action did not seem a promising avenue."[22] On the other hand, Risskov was well suited to studies of patients. In Danish hospitals, patients were consistently diagnosed "according to Kraeplinean traditions, and owing to the stability of the Danish population patients could be followed for many years." So Schou decided to focus on the use of lithium in patients.

Over the next five years, Schou continued to treat manic patients with lithium. He also carried out some basic pharmacological studies of lithium, examining in rats its effects on the kidney, heart, and other organs and the way the body absorbed and eliminated it. (His laboratory continued to do this sort of basic pharmacological research, focusing on lithium's side effects and their treatment.) Schou also started to keep a close eye, as he did for the rest of his life, on the research coming from other places.

Through the latter half of the 1950s, Schou wrote a dozen papers about lithium, reporting the results of his animal studies, the outcome of additional patients treated with lithium (most of these were in Danish), and a comprehensive review titled, "Biology and Pharmacology of the Lithium Ion."

Nonetheless, despite lithium's promise and Schou's persistent advocacy, the psychiatric community largely ignored lithium.

In 1958, the first International Congress of Neuropharmacology convened in Rome. This organization became, and has remained, the major international forum for imparting and discussing information about psychiatric drugs. It meets every two years and is now known—less than happily—as the Collegium Internationale Neuro-Psychopharmacologicum (CINP). For its first conference, in 1958, all the big names in the new science of psychopharmacology converged on Rome. The program included symposia and papers on the new antidepressants, tranquilizers, and antipsychotics. The conference proceedings ran to 720 pages. Lithium does not appear in the title of any paper. It came up only when Schou mentioned it as part of a "general discussion" at the end of the conference.

Well aware that his colleagues had shown little interest in lithium, Schou began his remarks with what he later called "a cry of despair and defiance." It turned out to be prophetic. He said: "On the chemotherapeutic firmament lithium is one of the smaller stars, and until now it may not even have been noticed by all psychiatrists. But its light appears unmistakable, and it may turn out to be more steady than that of several other of the celestial bodies which now shine so brightly."[23] Schou then spoke briefly about his work with lithium to date, reporting that he and his colleagues had given lithium to 157 patients with mania and that about 80 percent had responded favorably. He acknowledged the problem of lithium toxicity and pointed out that reduced sodium intake probably accounted for a good bit of it. He also noted that he and his colleagues had safely kept a number of patients on lithium for four years.

To Trautner, Noack, and Schou, it seemed clear that lithium warranted further study and that to ignore it was to needlessly prolong the suffering of those patients who could benefit from the drug. Nevertheless, lithium—this simple element—was largely ignored by both mainstream psychiatrists and drug researchers until well into the 1960s (the 1960 CINP meeting doesn't mention lithium at all, and the 1962 meeting relegates it to a comment by Schou on the last page of the proceedings).

Fortunately, a small number of professionals around the world remained intrigued by its potential. Throughout the early 1950s— soon after Cade's paper came out—a handful of psychiatrists in Australia, France, and England had started prescribing lithium. In France, lithium saw a flurry of attention in the early 1950s. Following Cade's lead, French psychiatrists gave lithium mostly to people with mania, but also to some with other states of excitement and psychiatric diagnoses. Between 1951 and 1955, 10 publications reporting the results of lithium treatment came out of France—more than the total publications from all other countries. None of these accounts entailed controlled, systematic research, none applied measurement of serum lithium levels, and some comprised just a few patients. Nonetheless, the results were promising. For the most part, patients with mania got better on lithium, in some cases showing remarkable and unprecedented improvement; and although the results were not entirely consistent, patients with schizophrenia and other ailments were less likely to improve.

It has never been clear why so soon after Cade's discovery lithium took off in France and, other than Australia, nowhere else.

The lithium historian Neil Johnson speculates that the popularity of mineral springs in France might have predisposed French psychiatrists to look favorably on a natural treatment—one, moreover, that was reputed to be a constituent of mineral springs. But even in France, the flurry of interest soon died out. Concerns over lithium's toxicity, a number of "accidents letaux" (lethal events), and the accepted effectiveness of ECT in mania contributed to the waning of interest. More than anything else, though, the advent in the early 1950s of the antipsychotic chlorpromazine—which among other things alleviated the excitement and other symptoms of mania—eclipsed lithium in France and elsewhere as well.

As for lithium's reception in Australia, by the mid-1950s, yet two more Australian doctors, in addition to Noack and Trautner, had described in published papers their experiences with lithium treatment. One was Bernard Glesinger, a psychiatrist at Claremont Hospital in Western Australia, who gave lithium to 104 patients and found that "the calming effect on maniacal, excited, hyperactive and restless patients was most satisfying and appreciable."[24] He provided a thorough review and discussion of lithium toxicity and side effects and, bucking the trend that started with Noack and Trautner, declared, "There is no necessity to measure or control lithium excretion by complicated chemical methods or to determine the plasma content. This refinement can be reserved for institutions with appropriate facilities. Lithium treatment can be carried out in any hospital safely and even at home under supervision."[25]

In a 1955 article published in the *Medical Journal of Australia*, the other Australian doctor who had begun to use lithium, Max Margulies, of Lachlan Park Hospital in Tasmania, reported that several years earlier he had started treating "maniacal" patients with lithium.[26] He had noted lithium's "objectionable" side effects, and to avoid them he used a lower lithium dose than the one in Cade's original report (10 grains of lithium citrate two or three times daily, rather than Cade's 20 grains). He didn't provide any details about these patients or their response to lithium, but he declared that "the results were often satisfactory; maniacal patients were very soon quietened and became in due time reasonably cooperative without wanting other sedatives, and some chronically ill patients could be restrained by a maintenance dose." He concluded that "the beneficial results in mania achieved with lithium alone have been confirmed." Margulies agreed with Ashburner that, while the fatal case reported by Roberts indicated the need for careful "medical supervision," it should not discourage further use of lithium.

Margulies's levelheaded appraisal of both the lithium research to date and his own experience with lithium in mania stands in contrast to the unrestrained therapeutic zeal he brought to other treatments, particularly, it seems, those he cooked up on his own. In his 1955 article "Suggestions for the Treatment of Schizophrenia and Manic-Depressive Patients," along with his account of lithium he gave a detailed description of "modified continuous narcosis," a treatment he devised that combined prolonged sleep induced by sedatives (at the time, a well-known treatment for an assortment of psychiatric ills) with—and this was Margulies's innovation—high doses of salicylates, the main chemical in aspirin. This regimen went on for seven days. Margulies allowed that after going through it patients were usually worse, but since several months later some of them seemed to improve, he thought he was onto something. "Modified continuous narcosis is sometimes useful after shock and insulin treatment have failed," he declared.

The intrepid Margulies had more than one string in his bow. In light of lithium's benefit in mania, he reasoned that if he combined lithium with a sedative, he could extend its benefit to patients with other conditions. So he proceeded to give some patients with schizophrenia and other psychoses both lithium and barbitone, a barbiturate widely used as a sleep aid. A few of these patients seemed to get better. Although Margulies acknowledged that the value of what he dubbed "combined lithium medication" was uncertain, he stressed that "some encouraging results should not be overlooked" and that combined lithium medication "should perhaps become the subject of large-scale investigations."

Margulies was hardly alone in having confidence in treatments that had no actual value; well into the middle of the twentieth century, well-meaning doctors routinely, and for the most part unwittingly, promoted all sorts of bunkum. They usually came with an elaborate, harebrained theory, they didn't actually work—there was simply no real evidence in support of them—and they were often dangerous. Thankfully, the treatments (other than lithium alone) that Margulies put forward in his 1955 article were less than compelling, and what happened in Tasmania stayed in Tasmania.

The fact that the psychiatric establishment was promoting and swearing by an assortment of useless therapies at the very time Cade was doing his lithium work puts Cade and his research in stark relief; it compels us to ask how Cade managed to come up with a therapy that was both so valid and so ahead of its time. Cade's interest in the details of the world around him—from the markings of magpies to animal scat to the floor of a Danish church—perhaps offer a clue. Although he certainly had theories about mental illness, those theories didn't seem to clutter his mind. He was first and foremost an observer and a relatively unbiased one. Perhaps more than anything else, straightforward unfettered observation allowed him to make his lithium discovery.

Once he made that discovery and duly published his report of it, Cade seemed to understand—and not be particularly troubled by—the delay of years before the psychiatric community recognized its importance. He recognized that the breakthrough had come from "an unknown psychiatrist."[27] And the fact that his landmark article appeared in the *Medical Journal of Australia*, a publication barely read outside of Australia and which some believed dealt chiefly with the treatment of snakebites, certainly did not help generate wide interest.

Yet Cade's observations inspired Trautner, Schou, Margulies, and several psychiatrists in England. One of the latter read an abstract of Cade's paper in the November 1949 issue of the *Digest of Neurology and Psychiatry*. Put out by the Institute of Living, a psychiatric hospital in Hartford, Connecticut, the *Digest* contained summaries of important articles and was distributed worldwide. Among the people who saw the abstract was Russell Murdoch Young, in 1949 the deputy medical superintendent of Parkside Hospital, in Macclesfield, England:

> I saw a summary of the original article in the *Australian Medical Journal* of 1948 or '49 . . . in the abstracts prepared for the Institute of Living, Hartford, Conn., and found a supply of effervescent lithium citrate on a back shelf of the Dispensary of Parkside Hospital. . . . I think this preparation had been recommended in the past as a health-giving mineral water but had not had much popularity. As instructed in the Australian article I gave the citrate in double the dose by weight recommended for the carbonate and was immediately converted by the dramatic way in which the manic symptoms were switched off in a few days in cases particularly of mild hypomania who were such a disruptive influence in a quiet ward. . . . There was no information about supervising blood levels and my half-hearted attempts to interest the pathologists in research failed, as I think they thought I was a mad psychiatrist playing with dangerous chemicals.
>
> I soon found that lithium seemed if anything, harmful in endogenous depressive states and the depressive phase of manic-depressive episodes, and though I used lithium to prevent recurrences in purely manic cases, unfortunately I never used it between attacks to prevent depressive relapses as has become regular practice since my retirement.
>
> The occurrence of several near disasters made me turn to phenothiazines when they appeared, but I never felt they were specific, and I continued to use lithium off and on when I felt it indicated.
>
> Unfortunately pressure of work, expanding services in the

community in the Manchester Region . . . prevented my publishing, though I spread the word by word of mouth to my colleagues in the early 'fifties. They also however were tempted by the more respectable and, to the drug firms, more profitable, phenothiazines, so I was rather a lone voice preaching in competition with mass advertising.[28]

Young's was indeed a lone voice—he was certainly one of the first in England to try lithium—but he was soon followed by David Rice, who, in the early 1950s, started giving lithium to patients at Graylingwell Hospital, a large psychiatric hospital in Chichester, Sussex. Rice, deputy medical superintendent at the hospital and, among his other accomplishments, a first-class cricketer, ended up writing the first British publication about lithium. Looking back 30 years, he recalled how he happened upon lithium:

> It all occurred almost by default, or accident. It was in about 1952–53 when I was in charge of the male side at Graylingwell Hospital, Chichester. I had at that time two particularly difficult and overactive patients with long hypomanic (manic) illnesses. In those days our pharmacological armamentarium was pretty limited. . . . I would have liked to give each of these chaps ECT but the relatives wouldn't allow it. We were pondering on what we could do when an Australian Registrar produced a scruffy crumpled sheet from the journal of the Australian Medical Association with Cade's article in it. I felt we had nothing to lose so decided to try it.[29]

Rice got encouraging results with the first two patients, and he went on to prescribe lithium to Graylingwell patients on a regular basis, particularly those with manic and hypomanic illness. In a 1956 *Journal of Mental Science* article, Rice described the effects of lithium in the first 58 patients.[30] He reported that of 37 patients with mania, 14 recovered and 20 improved. Of 16 patients with schizophrenia, 1 recovered and 5 improved. Rice acknowledged that he prescribed lithium "on clinical grounds . . . and without controlled experiment." Nonetheless, his observations were entirely consistent with those from Australia, France, and Denmark and provided additional confirmation of lithium's distinctive therapeutic properties.

Rice's major contribution to the development of lithium, though, was not his personal experience with it or the results of his study, but the people whom he inspired to use and research it. In 1956, at about the time that his paper turned up in the *Journal of Mental Science*, Rice moved eastward along the coast to Hailsham to be the medical superintendent at Hellingly Hospital, another large psychiatric hospital in Sussex. He told Ronald Maggs, a consultant psychiatrist at Hellingly who became a close colleague and friend, about his work with lithium. Captivated by Rice's account, Maggs tried it on one of his patients. "The results made such an impression on me," Maggs recalled, "that in spite of the development of the phenothiazines . . . I considered that this subject was worthy of further research."[31] He decided to follow up Rice's observations with a systematic clinical trial. Rice himself was not inclined to do further research with lithium. He had just taken over as medical superintendent and his administrative load didn't leave room for research; moreover, as he said, "I am afraid I haven't got a research mind." So he gladly left this next step to Maggs.

Maggs did have a penchant for research. He got himself a grant from the South-East Metropolitan Regional Hospital Board to support measurement of lithium levels and proceeded to carry out a meticulous, double-blind, "crossover" trial comparing lithium with placebo. Patients admitted to Hellingly Hospital in the midst of a manic episode and who were deemed suitable to be on the research protocol got two weeks of lithium and two weeks of placebo. Half the patients got lithium first and after two weeks of "rest" were then "crossed over" to placebo, and half got placebo first. Maggs drew on all the accoutrements of contemporary treatment research, including the use of established rating scales and advanced statistical methods to analyze the treatment results.

During lithium treatment, but not placebo, the symptoms of mania diminished substantially. Maggs's study, the most impeccably designed and controlled to date, showed unequivocally that lithium reduced the symptoms of mania and that its apparent benefit was not a result of wishful thinking or spontaneous improvement.

Maggs published the report of his study in 1963.[32] By that time, about two dozen articles describing the effects of lithium in mania were in psychiatric journals. With only one exception, these accounts showed that the majority of patients with mania improved on lithium. Yet of the studies published to that date, only those by Schou and Maggs had been at all "controlled." Maggs's study, along with Schou's, was instrumental in firmly establishing lithium as a treatment for mania. As the years went on, other controlled investigations confirmed their findings.

Maggs continued to do research both on lithium and on other psychiatric matters. As significant for the development of lithium treatment as his study of acute mania was his relationship with Alec Coppen, an eminent British psychiatrist and one of the founders of psychiatric drug treatment. They were both interested in the biochemistry of mental illness and in lithium therapy, and they collaborated on a number of research projects. In the late 1960s, Coppen decided to examine the idea, then very much in the air but controversial, that lithium could prevent episodes of both mania and depression. He organized a large definitive study that required a group of psychiatrists and several hospitals. Coppen invited Maggs to participate, and Maggs readily agreed. The results of this trial confirmed that lithium has a potent prophylactic effect in manic-depressive illness. These results, published in 1971, with Maggs as a coauthor, played a key role in establishing lithium's importance as a preventive agent—now its chief application—and helped set the stage for lithium's widespread use.

Rice's influence on lithium's fate did not end with Maggs. G. P. (Toby) Hartigan, a consultant psychiatrist at St Augustine's Hospital in Canterbury, learned of lithium from Rice's

1956 paper and in 1957, inspired by Rice's work, started giving lithium to patients with periodic attacks of mania and depression. Like others before him, Hartigan found that lithium prevented attacks of mood disturbance in most patients with either recurring mania or recurring attacks of both mania and depression. Hartigan also found—and this was new—that lithium stopped episodes of depression in people with recurring depression only. As we shall see, Hartigan's observations encouraged Schou and others to carry out the next round of lithium research. That research set the ball rolling for lithium to finally be recognized and applied as a unique prophylactic agent.

David Rice remained at Hellingly for the rest of his career. In 1960, a few years after his lithium paper appeared, he made his debut in first-class cricket (the highest level of the game). He was 46 at the time and the oldest first-class debutant in the British Isles since 1924. Rice continued to play top-rank cricket well into his 50s.

Despite the good—and in some instances astoundingly good—results that Schou and a few others saw with lithium, as the 1950s came to an end, the psychiatric community as a whole continued to ignore it. In a 1959 article that appeared in the journal *Psychopharmacologia*, Schou provided an update on lithium treatment with the paper "Lithium in Psychiatric Therapy: Stock-Taking after Ten Years." He had combed the world's psychiatric literature for accounts of manic patients treated with lithium and, as of early 1959, found 15 published reports, including Cade's and his own. The total number of treated patients, worldwide, came to 370. According to the authors of these reports, 304 of the patients (82 percent) had "improved." Schou acknowledged that this rate of improvement needed to be viewed cautiously; the authors varied in how they defined mania, how they defined improvement, and for how long they treated and observed the patients. Except for Schou's study, the lithium treatment was "uncontrolled," so it wasn't at all clear that lithium per se brought on the improvement.

Still, Schou noted the general agreement among the reports—

all but one found that the majority of manic patients improved with lithium—and felt that these combined observations suggested that lithium had a significant, albeit limited, role in treatment. "The main indication for lithium treatment," he wrote, "is the chronic manias, i.e. the cases with protracted or frequently recurring mania. This is a rather small group of patients, but very often these cases have proved resistant to most other therapies, and lithium treatment seems to offer the patients a very fair chance of either considerable improvement or total recovery, which they would not otherwise have had."[33]

Schou's claim for lithium, modest and reasonable as it was, fell on deaf ears. The second CINP Congress, in 1960, included no papers at all about lithium; and at the 1962 Congress, lithium came up only at the end when Schou made a comment about it in a general discussion at the close of the last symposium. The symposium was titled "Ten Years of Psychopharmacology: Critical Assessment of the Present and the Future." When Schou took the floor, he didn't mince his words:

Through its title and the communications so far given, this morning's discussion seems to be about to create the false historical myth that 1962 is the tenth anniversary of the psychopharmacological era. This, however, is neither true nor fair, because in 1949 the Australian, Cade discovered the therapeutic efficacy of lithium salts against manic phases of the manic-depressive psychosis.

There may be a number of reasons for the unjustified neglect of this drug during the years. One is its narrow spectrum of indication, namely the typical manias and especially the chronic ones; but a high specificity of a drug ought not to detract from the appreciation of it. Furthermore, it is known that lithium may under extreme conditions produce kidney damage; but we know a good deal about the mechanism of this toxic action and are accordingly able to prevent it effectively, and this is more than can be said about the toxic effects of most other psychotropic drugs. But the main reason for the neglect of lithium may be quite simply that lithium salts are so inexpensive that no commercial interests are involved. This drug has therefore completely lacked the publicity which is invariably given to drugs of higher money-earning capacity.[34]

In continuing to try and explain why lithium had been overlooked, Schou issued a warning about how bias can hamper innovation:

It is indeed conspicuous that lithium does not appear in any of the many general surveys, in spite of its therapeutic value being proved in a group of patients which was resistant to most other therapies. This may conceivably be due to mere ignorance, but such a suggestion is perhaps impolite. I would rather think that lithium is omitted from these schemes because it is chemically completely unrelated to any of the other drugs used in psychiatry. I am therefore in complete agreement with what Dr. Akimoto has just said. We must not let schemes and terminology, however beautiful and logically satisfying they may be, rule our thinking and obscure our observational powers. If, because it is easy or out of a desire for systematization, we adhere to a too categorical classification of drugs, we run the grave risk of distorting truth and of hampering scientific progress.[35]

By this time, Schou had been hammering away at lithium for 10 years. He had continued to give lithium to patients with mania (he tried it on some depressed patients as well, but abandoned that line of inquiry when the lithium didn't seem to work), he had kept on tracking the lithium findings coming from other places, and he had continued to document and research lithium's side effects and toxicity. Although the CINP and other congresses did not include formal papers or discussions about lithium, Schou spoke about it in informal gatherings at these conferences and elsewhere—to whoever would listen.

Notwithstanding Schou's insistence that lithium deserved a place in the avalanche of new psychiatric drugs, the fact is that had treating mania remained lithium's only use it would have never gotten off the ground. Chlorpromazine, which came on the scene in 1952, quickly surpassed lithium not only because it was promoted by drug companies, but also because in important ways it was a better treatment for mania. It usually takes about a week for lithium treatment to reduce symptoms of mania, whereas chlorpromazine, as well as the related drugs that came in its wake, improves these symptoms in hours. And chlorpromazine, although it has its own side effects, does not pose lithium's risk of serious toxicity and does not require blood level checks.

But lithium did get off the ground. In the early 1960s, at the same time that lithium seemed stalled as a treatment for mania, Schou began to spearhead an effort that ended up revealing an effect of lithium that dwarfed its use in acute mania and that, more than any treatment before or since, allowed people with manic-depressive illness to lead normal lives. Finally, the medical establishment would begin to give lithium the serious study that it deserved.

6

Prophylaxis Rex

IN 1960, Schou got letters from Toby Hartigan, in England, and Poul Baastrup, a psychiatrist working in Glostrup, Denmark. The letters arrived at about the same time and were about the same thing. Since 1957, both men had been treating patients with lithium (Hartigan learned of lithium from Rice's 1956 paper and Baastrup from a paper Schou had published in 1955). What prompted them to contact Schou was that they had found that lithium not only allayed the symptoms of mania, but could also prevent episodes of mania and, most importantly, could prevent episodes of depression as well. Schou was now recognized as the foremost lithium expert, and Hartigan and Baastrup wanted to know what he made of their observations, particularly lithium's unexpected ability to stop recurrent depression.

Hartigan had given lithium to 20 patients: 9 had episodes of just mania, 4 had periods of both mania and depression, and 7 had repeated bouts of depression. As in previous research, most of the patients with either mania alone or episodes of both mania and depression showed remarkable improvement; with few exceptions, lithium dispelled their manic symptoms and as long as they continued to take it seemed to prevent further episodes. There was nothing new in this. What was new came from Hartigan's decision to give lithium to patients with just recurrent depression. Hartigan was aware that the little research to date on lithium's use in depression suggested that it did not improve depressive symptoms, so rather than give lithium to patients in the midst of a depression, which seemed unlikely to be fruitful, he decided to see if lithium would prevent further depressions. Accordingly, he treated the patients' depressions with ECT, and when they had recovered, he started them on lithium. Hartigan treated 7 patients in this manner. They had suffered frequent attacks of severe depression, as many as three or four per year. With lithium treatment, 5 of these patients stopped having depressive episodes.

In 1959, Hartigan described his experiences with lithium, providing detailed accounts of several patients, in a paper he read to the Southeastern Branch of the Royal Medicopsychological Society. Hartigan's paper was noteworthy on several counts. Much of the early research on lithium, and certainly later research, focused on relapse rates and other statistics. In the reports of these studies, as is invariably the case in the reports of contemporary treatment studies, the victims of manic-depressive illness are numbers placed in one category or another. Hartigan's approach, like Cade's, was to portray in some detail what happened to particular patients when they got lithium:

> In relating my own experiences with the drug I have decided to describe in brief the case histories of certain individual patients. I have not concerned myself with the problem of proving or disproving the efficacy of the drug from a scientific standpoint as the numbers I have treated personally (only twenty) are insufficient for the purpose, and in any event . . . several large-scale trials, some even with acceptable controls, have already been carried out by others. . . . I hope, however,

that this anecdotal approach, though rightly much out of favour in academic circles, may be tolerated in as much as it may serve to indicate the types of patients who may be submitted to lithium therapy with a good prospect of a successful result.[1]

Indeed, Hartigan's paper offered a compelling account of how lithium can impact the life of a person with manic-depressive illness. It also showed that a scientific paper does not have to be mind-numbingly dreary.

Among the patients that Hartigan described was a 65-year-old woman who had been manic for several years: "She was interfering, vindictive, tactless, overbearing, inconsiderate, and altogether quite intolerable. She was extremely overactive, heedless of time, and she slept very little. Her husband, a long-suffering ex-hospital administrator who had been devoted to her, was on the brink of leaving her and she had alienated all her relatives and friends." Hartigan started her on lithium: "Within a month she had completely calmed down into a tranquil . . . state. On discharge she continued her reposeful mood and began to recover her interests in people and things, but she no longer shows any signs of her previous symptoms which had made her a domestic virago and a social menace. Her husband is the greatest lithium enthusiast in East Kent, and I have no doubt that it saved the marriage."[2]

Hartigan knew of Schou's interest in lithium and in August 1960 he wrote to him about what he had found: "I am venturing to send you a copy of a paper . . . that I read to a medical society last year. I do not think it publishable, but there are some observations which I think may be of interest to you, particularly those dealing with the prophylaxis of recurrent depression."[3] (Prophylaxis is the prevention of a disease.)

Schou replied immediately. He was interested indeed, thought that Hartigan's findings were important, and urged him to publish. It would be a pity, Schou wrote, "if these original observations and very convincing case histories were not brought to the attention of a larger group of psychiatrists."[4] Hartigan, though, had not published any papers previously and, aware of the scientific limitations of his findings, was not eager to pursue publication. In addition to believing—rightly—that his "anecdotal" (case history) approach was "out of favour in academic circles," he felt that the number of patients was too small for him to draw firm conclusions.

A year and a half later, in February 1962, Schou visited Hartigan in Canterbury and saw some of Hartigan's patients firsthand. He was struck by the fact that patients who had suffered repeated bouts of depression for many years had been free of depression for the two or more years they had been on lithium.

When he returned to Denmark, Schou immediately sent a letter to Hartigan thanking him for his hospitality, expressing, once again, his belief that lithium's apparent ability to put a stop to recurring depression was of great importance, and pressing him to publish: "I must say that I found the five cases presented very convincing," Schou wrote. "I have told my clinical colleagues about these patients, and we shall be on the look-out for patients who might fall in the category that seems to profit from preventive lithium treatment. May I once more urge you to publish your experiences; I consider them much too valuable to be hidden in a drawer."[5]

Hartigan, though, was in no rush to publish—he seemed happily impervious to the concept of "publish or perish"—and Schou's plea fell on deaf ears. Schou persisted. Seven months later, he sent another letter to Hartigan: "I know that you felt your material was too small to convince anybody. I do not agree with you there. If you have not yet done it, please consider again publishing a report. There comes a point where people may become suspicious if I continue referring to the 'unpublished observations' and 'personal communication' from G. P. Hartigan while this person himself remains silent!"[6]

Not hesitating to offer any advice that might get Hartigan into print, Schou added the specific suggestion that he send an account of his findings to Dr. Eliot Slater, editor of the *Journal of Mental Science*. Finally, Hartigan relented, and over the next few months, with Schou's help, he prepared a manuscript that Slater accepted for publication in the *British Journal of Psychiatry* (the new name for the *Journal of Mental Science*). The paper appeared in 1963 and was the first report to explicitly state that lithium could prevent severe depressive episodes.[7]

Hartigan also had a less formal role in lithium's emergence as a prophylactic agent. In 1961, Schou wrote to Hartigan asking if he had any additional information about lithium's effects in patients—and he let Hartigan know that his interest in lithium's benefits was not strictly academic. For 25 years, Schou's younger brother had suffered yearly episodes of depression. The depressions lasted several months, rendered him unable to work, and, despite hospital stays and treatment with ECT and drugs, would recur every spring. Schou wondered if lithium was worth a shot. Hartigan was encouraging. He told Schou that he thought "in your brother's case it should be well worth trying." Schou followed his suggestion and the results were nothing short of miraculous.

In an address he gave in 1981 upon receiving an honorary doctorate from the University of Aix-Marseille, Schou described what happened:

> The attacks usually lasted some months, and then disappeared, but they reappeared again and again, year after year, inevitably. Then, about 14 years ago, he was started on maintenance treatment with lithium, and since then he has not had a single depressive relapse. He still needs to take the medicine to keep the disease under control, but functionally he is a cured man. You will understand what such a change meant to himself and to his wife and children, and how much of a miracle it appeared to us in the family. Fear of the future has been replaced by confidence and new hope.[8]

As the years went by, a number of family members in addition to his brother got lithium treatment with good effect. Schou found it enormously gratifying that his research with lithium, in addition to improving the lives of millions and shedding light on the nature of manic-depressive illness, was also of direct benefit to his family.

But the fact that Schou had personal motives for investigating lithium turned out to be a double-edged sword. On the one hand, his brother's terrific response to lithium encouraged him to find out as much as he could about lithium and sustained him in his efforts to establish lithium as a treatment. On the other hand, as a consequence of his readiness to talk about his brother's excellent reaction to lithium, Schou was accused by some of being biased in favor of lithium, a "believer" rather than an objective scientist. This accusation ended up fueling a controversy about lithium's true benefit that went on for more than a decade. Psychiatrists on both sides of the Atlantic took sides. Although the controversy was largely resolved in the early 1970s, by that time it had degenerated into ad hominem attacks, and the resulting acrimony persisted for the lifetimes of the protagonists. Still, the very animosity of the argument had a silver lining; it pressed Schou and his colleagues to do the study that clarified lithium's unique value and led to its worldwide acceptance.

At about the same time that Hartigan began to treat patients with lithium, Poul Christian Baastrup, a Danish psychiatrist, started to give lithium to some of the patients admitted to the state mental hospital in Vordingborg, about 50 miles south of Copenhagen. Prompted by Schou's good results in patients with mania, Baastrup gave lithium to patients undergoing "exaltation," or excitement, most of whom were manic-depressive. Over two years he treated 56 patients. He confirmed Schou's observation that patients in the throes of the manic phase of manic-depressive illness were most likely to benefit from lithium; those with excitement resulting from other mental conditions did not appreciably improve. But Baastrup noticed something else as well:

As part of the trial, I conducted a follow-up examination on patients who had been discharged from hospital. After a short course of treatment at the out-patient clinic, they had been asked to stop taking lithium. There were two reasons for this examination: firstly, to make sure that patients did not continue to take lithium without the check-ups, and secondly, to see if lithium treatment had caused any undesirable late side effects or other complications. The result was hair-raising. Eight patients, all with a bipolar course, had continued to take lithium and two of them had even bestowed these "miracle pills" upon manic-depressive relatives. None of these people had had any kind of checkup, of course. Their reason for continuing the treatment in spite of our agreement was consistent: all of them said that continuous lithium treatment prevented psychotic relapse. These patients had had many psychotic episodes over a number of years (mean 12 years, range 3–25 years); from their own experiences they understood clearly their chances of relapse. I can still remember with what mixed and conflicting emotions I faced these eight patients. On the one hand, they had broken a definite agreement and exposed themselves to incalculable and indeterminate risks for which I was responsible. On the other hand, their gratitude at the results was so overwhelming and undeserved. But their claim, however convincing it might seem, could not be right? It did at least deserve to be refuted![9]

The suggestion that lithium—or any other drug, for that matter—could actually *prevent* attacks of mania and depression was totally unexpected, if not outlandish. (At this point, Baastrup did not know that Hartigan had found something similar.) Yet, like Cade before him, Baastrup grasped the potential implications of an unforeseen observation and proceeded to look into it. He started with a retrospective study. To find out if, as the reports of his patients suggested, treatment with lithium could in fact prevent bouts of mania and depression, Baastrup had to find patients who had been on lithium long enough to influence their pattern of relapses. Most of the patients he had treated had been on lithium for only short periods, nearly all having stopped treatment after they recovered, but 11 patients had stayed on lithium for a long time, at least three years. All had suffered frequent episodes of mania and depression before taking lithium, and all, after starting lithium, experienced a dramatic change in their illness. Most of them simply stopped having manic and depressive attacks altogether; a few had an occasional brief episode. Just as significant, when 5 patients stopped taking lithium, they all had recurrences; but when they started lithium again, they returned to their normal state and stayed that way.

At about the same time that Hartigan wrote to Schou about his lithium work, Baastrup also wrote to Schou, letting him know about his unexpected observations regarding lithium's preventive (prophylactic) effect. Schou was, needless to say, intrigued and encouraged Baastrup to pursue his findings and to publish his retrospective data. Like Hartigan, Baastrup was more a clinician than an academic psychiatrist and despite Schou's encouragement was in no rush to publish.

At first, Baastrup and Hartigan did not know that independently they had both found that lithium could prevent the frequent, intense mood disturbances of manic-depressive illness. But in due course Schou let them know of each other's work and sent Baastrup a copy of Hartigan's paper. In 1964, Baastrup finally got around to publishing a report describing the 11 patients. In it he mentioned Hartigan's related observations.[10]

Meanwhile, in a paper published in 1963, Schou proposed that lithium and some of the new antidepressants might be a novel class of psychiatric drugs, ones that not only relieved some of the symptoms of manic-depressive illness but treated all of its features, the disease itself. He named these drugs "mood-normalizers" or "normothymotics," from the Greek *thymos*, meaning "feelings, mind, spirit."[11]

For good reason, neither this concept nor the terms he suggested ever took off. The idea that lithium and antidepressants formed a similar class of drugs, specifically active against the manic-depressive disease, turned out to be incorrect; to begin with, the antidepressants did not actually relieve mania as some preliminary work cited by Schou had suggested. Schou later regretted writing this paper, realizing that it was more speculative than his usual fare and lacked solid support. Nonetheless, this paper contained a rather large kernel of truth.

In laying out his support for the concept of lithium as a mood-normalizer, Schou referred to both Baastrup's and Hartigan's observations regarding lithium's prophylactic effect. He also mentioned a patient in his original 1954 study for whom continuous lithium treatment had stopped outbreaks of both mania and depression. In the early 1950s, when they treated this man, Schou and his colleagues were not considering prophylaxis as one of lithium's benefits, and they did not pay particular attention to its preventive action in this patient. Now, in light of Hartigan's and Baastrup's related observations, Schou realized that this one patient may have revealed something important about lithium. In his paper about normothymotics, Schou, almost as an aside, mentioned that these drugs, lithium being the prime example, can both treat the symptoms of manic-depressive illness and prevent its characteristic attacks.

Hartigan, like others before and after him, speculated that lithium in some helpful way alters the chemistry of the brain. But as he stated in his 1959 paper, he did not see himself tackling the question of how lithium accomplishes what it does. Instead, he hoped his success with certain patients might at least point toward who would be helped most by lithium.

So, by 1964, several dozen accounts from around the world had confirmed that lithium quelled the symptoms of mania. And of greater import, it turned out, Hartigan, Baastrup, and Schou in three separate publications had explicitly raised the possibility that lithium could prevent bouts of mania and depression. Nonetheless, lithium had not yet caught the attention of mainstream psychiatry. Lithium's potential for harm and the availability of other drugs that could more quickly dispel manic symptoms made lithium's antimanic effects less than compelling. And the three reports documenting lithium's prophylactic effect, accurate and significant as they turned out to be, involved few patients and included no controls or other elements of systematic research. Understandably, perhaps, they drew little attention. Lithium was still the Cinderella of psychiatric drugs. Looking back at that time more than a decade later, Baastrup commented on the general reluctance to use lithium and particularly to give it continuously: "Both physicians to whom I had a near connection in my daily work and physicians working at the psychiatric clinic in the university of Copenhagen refused to use lithium; straightforward questions were answered in different ways—the treatment was too dangerous, the results published were incredible/untrustworthy/unreliable; the criticisms were never made publicly.[12]

This was about to change. Within three years, lithium came into its own and it fell to Baastrup, a methodical psychiatrist, plugging away and keeping careful watch over his patients, to start lithium on its final uphill battle.

Determined to find out if lithium really does put a stop to outbreaks of mania and depression, in 1960 Baastrup embarked on a prospective (going forward) study. He began this research at the same time as he was scouring hospital records for his retrospective inquiry, looking for patients who, for a variety of reasons, had been on continuous lithium treatment and seeing how they had fared. Although, as previously noted, his 11-patient retrospective study certainly seemed to confirm patients' testimonials regarding lithium's preventive ability, Baastrup knew that it would take a prospective analysis in which patients were systematically observed with and without lithium over an extended period to verify his observations.

Baastrup's prospective study went on for six and a half years. All of the patients were women admitted to Glostrup Psychiatric Hospital, on the outskirts of Copenhagen. During the study period, about 600 women came into the hospital with a diagnosis of manic-depressive psychosis, and about one-fourth of them got lithium. Baastrup selected 88 of these women for his study. He chose them on the grounds that before lithium treatment, they had suffered frequent episodes of mania, depression, or both (two or more episodes during one year or one or more episodes per year over two years). Baastrup observed each patient during about two years without lithium and then started long-term (at least one year) lithium treatment.

Schou and Baastrup had kept in touch since 1960, and although they lived and worked in different parts of the country, they decided to join forces on this prospective study. It was the first of many collaborative efforts. Baastrup treated and observed the patients, and Schou analyzed the data and wrote their joint paper. The paper appeared in the February 1967 issue of the *Archives of General Psychiatry*, a prestigious U.S. publication. In it, Baastrup and Schou showed that lithium had a striking prophylactic effect. Before lithium treatment, relapses had occurred on average every 8 months; during lithium treatment, only every 60 to 85 months. Before lithium, patients had spent on average 13 weeks per year in a psychotic state; during lithium, less than 2 weeks per year. Almost 80 percent of the patients had no relapses at all during lithium treatment. Baastrup and Schou concluded that "lithium is the first drug for which a clear-cut prophylactic action against one of the major psychoses has been demonstrated. We feel that lithium treatment can be of very considerable benefit to patients who suffer from a distressful and often disabling disease, and who are not easily or effectively helped by traditional therapies."[13]

Much of the world's psychiatric community agreed. Psychiatrists throughout Scandinavia and continental Europe found Baastrup and Schou's work convincing and started prescribing lithium. In short order, formal studies and the experiences of clinicians confirmed lithium's singular ability to prevent attacks of mania and depression. Recognition of lithium's prophylactic effect moved it to center stage in the treatment of manic-depressive illness.

Whereas the six CINP meetings between 1958 and 1968 contained no symposia on lithium and only two papers about it (both by Schou), at the seventh CINP meeting in 1970 the first symposium was titled "Clinical and Pharmacological Aspects of Lithium Therapy." The conference included 10 papers about lithium, and they came from all over—Belgium, Canada, Czechoslovakia, Denmark, Ireland, the United States. Over the next decade, the use of lithium mushroomed, research on it escalated, and its value became firmly established.

Yet in the late 1960s, despite its embrace by much of the world, psychiatrists in the United States and Britain were skeptical. The U.S. reluctance to accept lithium rested on several grounds: the lithium salt substitute debacle was still fresh in the minds of many, and neither the psychiatric community nor the FDA wanted to step again into those waters; despite the proliferation of new psychiatric drugs, psychoanalytic concepts and therapy still dominated U.S. psychiatry, and many psychiatrists considered any drug treatment, lithium included, to be at best an adjunct to psychotherapy; and unlike other new psychiatric drugs, lithium had no advocates in the powerful pharmaceutical industry.

Nonetheless, starting in the early 1960s, a handful of U.S. psychiatrists began treating patients with lithium and doing lithium research. Their persistence and the encouraging findings from their research convinced the wider psychiatric community to use lithium; and finally, in 1970, the FDA gave it official approval.

Notable among the people who got the lithium ball rolling in the United States were Sam Gershon and Ronald Fieve. In 1959, Gershon got a Pfizer Fellowship, which brought him from Australia to the University of Michigan for one year to work in a schizophrenia research program. While there, he filled in his Michigan associates on lithium's benefits and treated about 20 patients with lithium. He also gave lectures about lithium at the National Institute of Mental Health and elsewhere. And during that year, he and Arthur Yuwiler, a Michigan colleague, wrote a paper titled "Lithium Ion: A Specific Psychopharmacological Approach to the Treatment of Mania," which in 1960 appeared in the *Journal of Neuropsychiatry*, a U.S. publication. The paper summarized the available information on lithium's effects in psychiatric patients and covered in considerable detail how lithium should be prescribed and its toxicity avoided. It was the first U.S. publication on lithium and as such introduced American psychiatrists to this promising but largely unheard of new treatment.

After his year in Michigan, Gershon returned to Melbourne for one year and then in 1963 emigrated to the United States. He brought his enthusiasm for lithium and his considerable lithium know-how with him. In 1965, he became director of the Neuropsychopharmacology Research Unit at New York University. There he established a lithium clinic and research programs devoted to lithium and bipolar disorder. Gershon and his collaborators did a series of studies that supported lithium's specificity for the treatment of bipolar disorder, identified some of lithium's important side effects, including interference with the activity of the thyroid gland, and compared lithium with other psychiatric drugs.

Through both his own research and the research he inspired, as well as his warm relationships with both junior colleagues and the movers and shakers in American psychiatry, Gershon had a major impact on lithium's acceptance in the United States. His energy and infectious enthusiasm, along with his scientific acumen, made him an influential advocate for lithium. As Burt Angrist, one of the many whom Gershon mentored, put it: "I liked Sam immediately. The first qualities that struck me were his cordiality, utter lack of pretense, generosity with his time, and wonderfully 'goofy' sense of humor." Gershon's research unit, Angrist said, "was a place where his enthusiasm, humor and kindness were palpable to us all. A group of unusually odd characters, united in their loyalty to Sam, became friends and worked with an enthusiasm that I have not seen before or since."[14]

Gershon stayed at NYU for 15 years and then went on to senior posts at several other medical schools. He served on the American Psychiatric Association's Task Force on Lithium, convened in 1969, which advised the FDA on the efficacy and safety of lithium therapy. In 2006, Gershon retired from his position as vice president for research at the University of Pittsburgh Medical Center and moved to Miami. Six months later, the new chairman of the Department of Psychiatry at the University of Miami asked him to join the department as vice chairman of academic affairs. Gershon did so and remained in that position for the rest of the decade, finally retiring once again at age 86.

Among his raft of scholastic endeavors, Gershon was the editor-in-chief of *Bipolar Disorders*, an international journal devoted to basic and clinical studies, from 1999—the year he founded it—to 2017, when at age 89 he turned over the reins. Now age 90 and according to him "fully retired" and "leading the life of an elderly gentlemen," Gershon chairs data and safety monitoring boards in Pittsburgh and Canada, groups of experts responsible for overseeing research on new treatments. He also contributes regularly to a widely read psychiatric blog and a website devoted to the history of psychiatric drug treatment. He writes about many topics, including, of course, lithium.

In 1958, Ronald Fieve was in the midst of his psychiatric training at New York's Columbia University and was becoming increasingly disenchanted with his chosen field; he found the prevailing psychoanalytic approaches less than fully convincing: "I rapidly became frustrated and disillusioned with lack of results in my neurotic out-patients when I did my utmost to provide insight into their problems using what was then called 'talking cure.' With my in-patients, months of psychoanalytically-oriented psychotherapy did little to alleviate the symptoms of mania, depression or schizophrenia."[15] Fieve was about to throw in the towel. He told the chairman of the Psychiatry Department, Lawrence Kolb, that he didn't think he belonged in psychiatry, was more medically oriented, and felt he should return to internal medicine. (Fieve had done a year of internal medicine residency and then switched to psychiatry.)

Kolb had just returned from a conference in Australia where he had heard about Cade's lithium work, and he encouraged Fieve to look into the reports coming out of Australia and Denmark about this new treatment. As it happens, Heinrich Waelsch, a professor of biochemistry at Columbia and chief of psychiatric research, was also interested in lithium. His interest arose out of his direct contact with Mogens Schou. Waelsch and Schou had stayed in touch since the early 1950s, when Schou spent a year as a fellow in Waelsch's laboratory. Waelsch learned firsthand of Schou's experience with lithium during a visit with him in Denmark, and he returned to New York eager to work with it.

So, with Kolb encouraging him and paving the way and Waelsch providing biochemistry expertise and laboratory resources, Fieve, still a psychiatric resident, began treating manic-depressive patients with lithium. He went on to carry out systematic studies of lithium as a treatment for both manic and depressive episodes. These studies confirmed lithium's value in the treatment of mania and also verified its lack of effectiveness as a remedy for acute depression.[16] In the mid-1960s, Fieve started reporting the results of his research at U.S. psychiatric meetings and in the widely read *American Journal of Psychiatry*. His studies were the first systematic controlled lithium studies in the United States, and they helped generate interest among U.S. psychiatrists in a treatment that was still largely unknown.

Lithium research got a boost when in 1964 Kolb asked Fieve to set up a special research ward devoted to biochemical studies of manic-depressive patients who were on lithium. Kolb asked John A. Talbott, then the chief psychiatry resident at Columbia, to help get the ward under way and manage it. In one of the twists of fate that seem to arise with uncanny regularity in the lithium story, Talbott was the son of John H. Talbott, the physician who had played a key role 15 years earlier in both the lithium salt substitute debacle and the development of lithium level measurement. Yet John A. Talbott didn't know of his father's role in the development of lithium treatment until I mentioned it to him during an interview in 2017. Given his own immersion in early lithium research, Talbott was flabbergasted that he had not known of his father's connection to lithium. Recalling the early lithium research at Columbia, Talbott said: "Ron Fieve, Stan Platman and I set up the first lithium ward. I don't know if it was in the world, but at least in America. During all this time that we were setting up this lithium lab and the ward and patients and everything else, I never heard a word about my father, not a word."[17]

In 1966, Fieve went on to set up a lithium clinic at the New York State Psychiatric Institute, part of Columbia, originally to provide follow-up care for patients who had left the lithium ward. He also began treating patients with lithium in his private practice. Then in 1973, with a donation from a wealthy patient, Fieve bought a townhouse on 57th Street in tony midtown Manhattan and started the Foundation for Depression and Manic Depression. It provided psychiatric care for patients with these disorders, offered education and training, and carried out research with a particular focus on the treatment of these illnesses with lithium. Although Fieve passed away in early 2018, the foundation is still supported with private donations and remains focused on lithium research.

As the founder and director of three facilities devoted to lithium treatment and research, facilities that reached from academic and public psychiatry to the private sector, Fieve, in the 1970s, became a one-man sponsor and source of information about lithium. His scientific bent and grasp of treatment research, in combination with his entrepreneurial flair and showmanship, made him a singular advocate for lithium. He influenced and educated his psychiatric colleagues, the general public, and the FDA.

In 1964, having heard of Fieve's work with lithium, Joseph Tupin and his psychiatrist colleagues in Galveston, Texas, sent him a patient, a college professor who, despite treatment with massive doses of Thorazine (chlorpromazine), a potent tranquilizer and antipsychotic drug, remained confined in a Texas state mental hospital, uncontrollably manic. He was simultaneously writing 10 books and 40 research papers. After several weeks in New York, getting lithium from Fieve, the man calmed down. He returned to Texas "completely normal in mood and behavior."[18] Tupin and his colleagues, amazed by this man's recovery after many years of severe mood swings, filed an Investigational New Drug (IND) application with the FDA, requesting permission to investigate lithium. They began treating manic patients with lithium and reporting their results. And so lithium moved west.

Throughout the 1970s, Fieve took it upon himself to increase the public's awareness of manic-depressive illness and its successful treatment with lithium. He appeared on countless TV talk shows extolling the benefits of lithium, and in 1975 he published *Moodswing*, a book about manic depression. It became a bestseller and sold over a million copies. In 1973, he invited Joshua Logan, the celebrated playwright, director, and producer—and his patient—to appear with him on a televised AMA symposium about depression. Logan spoke candidly and in detail about his struggles with mania and depression and about his recuperation with lithium. He went on to become a spokesperson for the value of lithium, and he and Fieve formed a persuasive duo on the talk show circuit. When in 1973 they appeared with Barbara Walters on NBC's *Today*, the station was flooded with phone calls for weeks afterward.

For the rest of his life, Fieve directed the Foundation for Depression and Manic Depression and was actively involved in treating patients and conducting lithium research. He died from heart failure on January 2, 2018, at age 87. Just hours before his death, he evaluated a patient via telemedicine.

By the late 1960s, drums were beating in several quarters for the FDA to authorize lithium. (Regulatory agencies around the world had approved it years earlier.) The October 1968 issue of the *American Journal of Psychiatry* featured a special section on lithium comprising a dozen articles. In 1969, the American Psychiatric Association set up a task force on lithium to assess the value of lithium therapy and the advisability of having it available for general prescription use. Along with Sam Gershon, the task force included Ron Fieve, Joe Tupin, and several others. At that time, the FDA classified lithium as an Investigational New Drug, so it was not readily available. A psychiatrist who wanted to use it legally had to request permission from the FDA by going through the laborious process of filing an IND. As the 1960s drew to a close and word about lithium's value spread, hundreds of psychiatrists inundated the FDA with lithium INDs. These applications were ostensibly to conduct studies of lithium, but in fact most of the psychiatrists submitting them simply wanted to acquire lithium so they could give it to their patients. In addition, an untold number of psychiatrists, in what has been described as a "lithium underground," got hold of lithium and prescribed it without bothering to seek permission.

Paul Blachly, a professor of psychiatry at the University of Oregon Medical School, said publicly that despite the FDA's ban, he had arranged for a local drug manufacturer to place reagent-grade lithium into capsules and had been giving it to patients. He believed that physicians have a moral obligation to disobey the FDA when, as in the case of lithium, it forbids the prescription of a drug that is useful and safe. Regardless of the FDA's position, Blachly wrote, "the modern, scientifically-trained physician has a deeply-rooted fundamental right, indeed responsibility, to use that treatment which he feels is best."[19] Blachly, who recognized early on the importance of lithium and coauthored a comprehensive monograph about it, excoriated the FDA for its continued ban of lithium. In a stream of pointed correspondence, he challenged the FDA to justify its prohibition; and he appealed to senators and representatives to get the FDA to change its stand.

Gershon, Tupin, Fieve, and a handful of their colleagues lobbied the National Institute of Mental Health, the FDA, and anyone else who would listen to get lithium available for general use. The problem was that lithium fell outside the usual pathway for drug approval. Typically, a new drug is synthesized by a pharmaceutical company, the company takes out a patent on it, and then the company conducts tests to show that the drug is safe and effective. Lastly, the company files a New Drug Application (NDA) with the FDA, requesting permission to manufacture and market the drug. The dilemma around lithium was that since it didn't require synthesis—the corner pharmacist can provide the medicine by getting some inexpensive lithium salt from a chemical supply house and putting it into a capsule—and there was nothing to patent, there was little profit to be had. No drug firm clamored to produce it. So who or what would file an NDA?

As pressure for lithium to be more accessible continued to mount, the American College of Neuropsychopharmacology, an association of psychiatric drug researchers, considered filing an NDA in its own name so that lithium could be legally prescribed. This became unnecessary when, finally, three drug companies submitted applications to the FDA for approval of lithium. In April 1970, with guidance from the lithium task force, the FDA authorized lithium for the treatment of manic episodes. By then, 49 countries had already approved lithium. The United States was the 50th. Nathan Kline, a pioneer in psychiatric drug research and a major advocate for lithium, speculated that many of the FDA staff were eager to grant the approval simply to avoid having to process the continuing flood of IND applications from individual psychiatrists. In 1974, mainly on the basis of a large U.S. study that documented lithium's preventive value, the FDA extended its approval of lithium to include prophylactic treatment of manic-depressive illness.

Through the 1970s, following lithium's approval by the FDA and with several controlled studies having confirmed that it both alleviates mania and puts a stop to episodes of mania and depression, U.S. psychiatrists took on lithium. By the end of the decade, it was widely used; it had transformed the treatment of manic-depressive illness and drastically improved its prognosis.

Still, acceptance of lithium came more slowly in the United States than in continental Europe and Scandinavia. It wasn't just lingering concerns about lithium's dangers from the salt substitute debacle, although that played a part. During and shortly after World War II, a number of European psychoanalysts had emigrated to the United States, including some who had been in Freud's inner circle. They, along with America's general receptiveness to psychoanalysis, essentially moved the hub of psychoanalysis from Vienna to the United States. Well into the 1980s, psychoanalytic concepts dominated American psychiatry. For many psychiatrists, some form of psychoanalytic therapy was the gold standard for treating almost all conditions of the mind, including severe depression and the depressive phase of manic-depressive illness. Psychiatric drugs were considered, at best, an accessory to bona fide treatment. More than a few psychiatrists of that era believed that psychiatric drugs interfered with the therapy process or provided relief of symptoms that was not genuine or lasting.

I was a psychiatry resident in the late 1960s and early 1970s and, as was the case in most university medical centers, my teachers were psychoanalysts. Although antidepressant drugs had been around for 10 years and ECT for more than 30, I was instructed to treat depressed patients in line with the prevailing psychoanalytic formulation: depression results from anger turned inward. My fellow trainees and I spent hours trying to get our patients to talk about their anger. We were encouraged to avoid or minimize the use of psychiatric drugs, and ECT was a last resort.

Now the tables have turned; the approach I was taught would amount to malpractice. Today we view mental disorders as brain diseases; psychiatric drugs are the mainstay of treatment, and few psychiatrists practice psychotherapy.

Although lithium and other drugs that prevent attacks of mania and depression—so-called mood stabilizers—are now an indispensable part of psychiatric treatment, skepticism about lithium's value and lingering concerns about its dangers persisted for several years following FDA approval. In 1976, *Maude*, a popular TV sitcom, devoted two episodes to manic-depressive illness. Norman Lear, *Maude*'s producer, flew Nathan Kline to Los Angeles for a week to consult on the show. Kline had a huge and lucrative private practice in New York, and in addition to being an innovative psychopharmacologist and early promoter of lithium, he was brilliant and flamboyant in about equal parts. Following Kline's advice, the original script had a psychiatrist, whom Maude consults because of her abrupt mood swings, diagnose manic-depressive illness. The psychiatrist explains that this disorder is a "physical" problem, a "chemical imbalance in the blood," usually easy to control with lithium, and he proceeds to treat her with lithium successfully.

The advance publicity for the episodes mentioned Maude's good response to lithium. Although the show's reference to lithium was realistic and judicious, in 1976 lithium was still on shaky ground, and a number of psychiatrists, covering the spectrum from analysts to psychopharmacologists, objected to lithium's positive portrayal. The ensuing controversy got a good deal of press coverage. Lithium is dangerous, some declared. Sam Gershon, quoted in a *New York Times* piece on the show, said, "I have no serious reservations about lithium when used properly, but manic-depression is not a common disease, and that's what it should be used for."[20] He and others worried that lithium's favorable depiction on *Maude* could encourage a "massive outpouring of demand," a public clamor for lithium from people expecting to be cured of all sorts of psychiatric problems, including "simple cases of the blues." And some psychiatrists took exception as well to the depiction of a grave psychiatric problem in the unserious atmosphere of a sitcom.

Lear had wanted to do these shows, including the bit about lithium, as a public service. His wife at the time, on whom the character of Maude was loosely based, suffered from manic depression and had done well on lithium. Lear proceeded to read about lithium, and as he pointed out in the midst of the controversy over the pending episodes, he had consulted with Kline and other experts to make sure that the show treated the subject accurately and responsibly. Nonetheless, in light of the disapproval coming from psychiatric circles, the show's scriptwriters substituted "proper medication" for "lithium."

Nathan Kline didn't give up easily. When he learned that the original script had been altered to remove mention of lithium, he set up a meeting with Ron Fieve; he had heard that one of Fieve's patients was high up at CBS and hoped that Fieve would prevail on this patient to get lithium back in the show. According to David Dunner, a psychiatrist who worked alongside Fieve throughout the 1970s, Kline and Fieve were high-profile competitors.[21] Both were entrepreneurial, flamboyant, and gifted scientists. Both campaigned hard for lithium, and both had practices, as actress Patty Duke put it, "crammed with Wall Street tycoons and Hollywood producers."[22] If you were rich, well connected, and bipolar—and could get to Manhattan—you went to either Kline or Fieve. There was no love lost between the two. ("We never hit if off that great," Fieve said 50 years later, in what is probably an understatement.[23]) In Dunner's nine years with Fieve, the meeting about *Maude* is the only time he recalls the two men getting together. Despite Kline's maneuvering, *Maude* went on without lithium. Still, Kline's foray into prime-time television was not a total loss. Although he didn't get the lithium he so valued into the script, the *Maude* show did put in a plug for *From Sad to Glad*, Kline's book for the general public about depression.

Over the next few years, mainstream American psychiatry, including psychoanalysts, fully embraced lithium therapy, recognizing both its safety and its indisputable value in putting a stop to attacks of mania and depression. Lithium's high regard in the psychiatric community is of a piece with its now positive portrayals in fiction, in nonfiction memoirs of bipolar patients, and on TV. In TV land, as in the real world, times have changed since *Maude*. The hugely popular contemporary espionage thriller *Homeland*, which had its television debut in 2011 and finished its seventh season in 2018, features Carrie Mathison, a brilliant CIA agent played by Claire Danes, who is manic-depressive and handles her job and personal life well—as long as she stays on lithium. When, out of neglect or because she decides it's no longer necessary, Carrie stops taking her lithium, she spirals into a manic episode, talking nonstop, insisting on pursuing far-fetched plans, and prowling the city for one-night stands.

In *Homeland*, lithium, far from being unmentionable, is one of the key supporting players. "It keeps me safe and sane," Carrie confesses to a fellow agent. The show's depiction of her manic attacks, the crushing depressions that follow them, and lithium's critical role in her life have been praised for their authenticity by both health professionals and similarly affected patients.

Hannah Jane Parkinson, a journalist with bipolar disorder, believes that the depiction of Carrie's manic depression in *Homeland* is reminiscent of her experience with the illness. She points to how Carrie's rapid thoughts and surplus of ideas during manic episodes often result in significant breakthroughs in her work. Parkinson notes that the negative features of mania are also depicted: "lack of risk inhibition, the elusiveness of sleep, promiscuity, alienation of friends and family, drinking." Observing that we live "in a world in which mental health stigma is still devastating," Parkinson concludes, "that the lead protagonist of one of the most popular global television shows . . . is intelligent, charming, attractive and just happens to have a serious mental illness, is nothing short of a triumph."[24]

SEVERAL DECADES before *Homeland*—and even before *Maude*—while Kline, Fieve, Gershon, and Blachly were laboring to get lithium accepted and available in the United States, Schou and a group of British psychiatrists got into a battle about lithium, a malicious and prolonged one, that delayed acceptance of lithium therapy in the United Kingdom and to this day is not fully resolved.

The trouble started in 1966 at a small psychiatric meeting in Göttingen, Germany, organized by the chair of the local Department of Psychiatry. Schou was invited to the meeting, as was Michael Shepherd, a rising star at London's formidable Maudsley Hospital and Institute of Psychiatry and a staunch—some might say unyielding—advocate for the application of rigorous scientific methods to psychiatry research. He had pioneered clinical trial methods and was a stickler when it came to applying them. Shepherd had a dazzling intellect but was shy and socially awkward. He didn't suffer fools gladly, and it didn't take much to evoke his scorn.

At the Göttingen meeting, Shepherd gave a talk about the principles of clinical evaluation and the importance of using rigorous clinical trial methods—placebo controls, blinded evaluation, and so forth. Then Schou got up to speak, and he presented the results of the prophylaxis study that he had carried out with Baastrup. The findings were striking; manic-depressive patients treated with lithium fared much better during a year or more of lithium treatment than they had in the two years before starting lithium. The study had not yet been published, and Schou anticipated that his colleagues at the meeting would be pleased to learn that lithium not only relieved mania, but could also prevent attacks of mania and depression.

Impressive as the results were, Schou and Baastrup's study had not used the sort of rigorous research methods advocated by Shepherd, methods that, thanks to Shepherd and a handful of others, were quickly becoming the standard approach to treatment research; among other things, Baastrup and Schou had not used placebo controls, and neither the patients nor those treating them were "blinded" to the treatment in progress.

In recalling the meeting 30 years later, Shepherd had no trouble remembering his consternation:

 Schou got up and he was billed to talk about lithium in affective disorders. I expected to hear about mania and what not. But what I got for the first time was this view that lithium was everything, that it prevented the disease, that it treated the disease etc. I remember it very well because I was sitting at the back of the hall and one of the Germans wrote me a little note and he said "this man is contradicting everything you've just been saying." As I listened I could see that this was absolutely true. I remember also thinking, "I hope to heaven that I'm not asked to participate in the discussion." I tried to make myself inconspicuous . . . but of course I was asked as a guest.[25]

Recalling his comments on Schou's talk, "I tried to be as tactful as I could," Shepherd maintained. Nevertheless, he stated in no uncertain terms that the evidence Schou put forward was not good enough to conclude that lithium prevents bouts of mania and depression. As Shepherd further recalled:

> Afterwards Mrs Schou took me aside and said "you know, you were very severe and you've upset Mogens very much." I said "well what have I done" and she said "you've implied that what he was saying was doubtful and that more evidence was needed" and I said "well surely that is the case," still not fully realizing. Then he came and joined us and I can remember it very clearly. I realized that I was in the presence of a believer—somebody who knew. There were a lot of them about in most fields. He told me that a relative had been ill and that he was taking it and that really there ought to be a national policy in which everybody could get lithium. Because he has this jovial manner I wasn't altogether certain that he was serious but then I realized he was.[26]

Schou saw the point of Shepherd's methodological criticisms. He acknowledged that his research approach to the prophylaxis question had not been ideal, but he did not feel, as Shepherd did, that his admittedly flawed methods rendered the results worthless. Still, Schou thought that the disagreements between him and Shepherd about clinical trial methods and data analysis were legitimate matters for discussion. "Critical debate is what science thrives on and should at all times be welcomed," Schou declared.[27]

What Schou found inexcusable, though, were Shepherd's insistence that Schou had personal—and questionable—motives for studying lithium and that he lacked proper scientific objectivity. Both Shepherd and Schou trace the beginning of what became one of the most rancorous disputes in the history of psychiatric research to the Göttingen meeting. As bitter as it was, their wrangling was not unique. To the layperson, medical researchers may be shining examples of people dedicated solely to unearthing the truth—and nothing else; but they are in fact at least as prone to emotional reactions as everyone else. They jockey for position, especially when it comes to high-stakes discoveries. In the 1980s, for example, a team of French scientists led by Luc Montagnier battled an American research team led by Robert Gallo over which one of them deserved credit for discovering the HIV virus. It took until 1987 for a truce of sorts to be reached, and that occurred only because the heads of their two countries announced that Montagnier and Gallo would both be recognized as having discovered the virus (and that both research teams and their governments would share the royalties from a test for HIV). Though Shepherd may not have been driven by an urge to compete with Schou, he did believe that only he, not Schou, could perceive the truth. What could have been an academic debate about how to conduct lithium research became a personal feud.

Recalling that meeting in Göttingen 40 years later, Schou wrote, "When Shepherd . . . heard me lecture about prophylactic lithium treatment in Germany and express gratification with the results he immediately perceived me as a naïve and biased 'believer'. The crucial point seems to have been reached when I told how my brother, who for twenty-five years had had depressions every spring, stopped having recurrences when he was given lithium. Shepherd obviously found that this was the final testimony of my folly and subjectivity."[28]

Schou's memory of the Göttingen meeting differed a bit from Shepherd's; in a 1996 interview, Schou characterized as "pure invention" Shepherd's claim that Mrs. Schou came up to Shepherd and complained that he had upset her husband. But both men agreed that their quarrel began in Göttingen.

Soon after the Göttingen meeting, the paper reporting Baastrup and Schou's prophylaxis results appeared in the prominent *Archives of General Psychiatry* under the title "Lithium as a Prophylactic Agent: Its Effect against Recurrent Depression and Manic-Depressive Psychosis." In concluding the paper, Baastrup and Schou didn't hedge their bets. They wrote that "lithium is the first drug demonstrated as a clear-cut prophylactic agent against one of the major psychoses."

Shepherd and his Maudsley colleagues looked with disdain on treatments that were not supported by firm evidence and on research—as was the case with Baastrup and Schou's—that did not adhere to rigorous methods. They also prided themselves on skewering psychiatric myths; a decade earlier, the Maudsley group had rightly debunked insulin coma as a treatment for schizophrenia. Baastrup and Schou's study had undeniable flaws. Yet largely as a result of this study—and Schou's advocacy—the belief that lithium was a prophylactic agent had gained fairly wide acceptance, and lithium started to be used for this purpose throughout Scandinavia and continental Europe. This was simply too much for Shepherd. He prevailed upon Barry Blackwell, a younger colleague at the Maudsley, to scrutinize and appraise the Danish study, and together they wrote a critique—some would say an attack—that appeared in the May 4, 1968, issue of *The Lancet*. They titled it "Prophylactic Lithium: Another Therapeutic Myth?"

Blackwell and Shepherd found fault with everything from the way Baastrup and Schou had selected patients (some, they argued, may not have had the recurrent episodes typical of manic-depressive illness) to the statistics they applied and the criteria they used for prophylaxis (since the study was not placebo-controlled, what looked like a preventive action of lithium might have been spontaneous remission, and the apparent fall in relapse rate a chance fluctuation). Most damning of all, they argued that the results were unreliable because Baastrup and Schou were biased in favor of lithium: according to Blackwell and Shepherd, the investigators were "enthusiastic advocates" for lithium therapy and had been so for several years. Because the study was "open," not controlled or blinded, Baastrup and Schou knew when a patient was and was not taking lithium, and Blackwell and Shepherd maintained that this knowledge, along with their belief in the value of lithium, had affected the way they evaluated and managed the patients. "A clinician committed to the ideal of 'prophylaxis,'" Blackwell and Shepherd wrote, "will be prepared to manipulate dosage and give adjunctive outpatient support to forestall admission, itself the main criterion of success or failure (of lithium therapy)."

Blackwell and Shepherd concluded that Baastrup and Schou's methods were shoddy and their results unconvincing, if not total rubbish: "The criteria for selection of patients and for prophylaxis are not rigorous enough, and . . . the results were subject to faulty evaluation and observer bias." Given the fact that there had been a rapid increase in the use of lithium as a prophylactic agent, Blackwell and Shepherd stressed the need for a properly controlled clinical trial to verify (or not) lithium's value. Baastrup and Schou's study, in their view, had fallen far short.

Baastrup and Schou promptly fired off an article to *The Lancet* in which they reviewed the methods and results of their study and responded in detail to Blackwell and Shepherd's criticisms.[29] The key flaw in their study, according to Blackwell and Shepherd, had been their failure to compare lithium with a placebo or some other treatment. In their original paper, Baastrup and Schou had provided the rationale for doing this sort of "open" study rather than a more conventional and methodologically rigorous placebo-controlled, blinded study. Because they had observed a "striking prophylactic action of lithium" in Baastrup's first group of patients, they thought it would be cruel—and unethical—to withhold lithium from some patients, giving them instead a placebo or the traditional (and in most cases ineffective) therapy and thereby subjecting these patients to the devastation of relapses. Further, Baastrup and Schou contended that they didn't need to divide the patients into two groups, one getting lithium and one not, to demonstrate a prophylactic effect. They assumed, with reasonable justification, that patients would sustain the rate of relapse they experienced during the period without lithium. Thus, a prophylactic effect could be adequately evaluated, they thought, by using patients as their own "controls," tracking the rate of relapse before and after lithium.

In their rebuttal, Baastrup and Schou dismissed out of hand the Brits' implication that psychological effects of the treatment—

increased attention to patients, the investigators' enthusiasm—
contributed to the apparent success of lithium. There was simply
no reason to believe, they declared, that either suggestion or these
sorts of strictly psychological factors could alter the course of so
serious a disease.

As for the charge that their enthusiasm for lithium had influenced the way they evaluated patients, causing them to minimize,
or even forestall, relapses during lithium treatment, Baastrup and
Schou countered, as they had indicated in their original paper,
that a flare-up of symptoms was defined as a relapse only when
it was sufficiently severe to require hospital admission or regular
supervision in the home. In their rebuttal, they pointed out that
since "decisions concerning those measures were not made by
us," the judgment of relapse was "uninfluenced by possible investigator bias."

In wrapping up, Baastrup and Schou wrote, "Our study on
lithium prophylaxis was the first of its kind. It could have had a
different design and possibly a better one. But even a design that is
short of the ideal may, in addition to the advantage of being practically feasible, constitute useful information if the study succeeds
in proving its point beyond a reasonable doubt."

The battle was on and it went viral, 1960s style. *The Lancet* is
a highly regarded, influential medical journal based in Britain but
read all over the world. It is one of the oldest and best-known
medical periodicals. Blackwell and Shepherd's blast and Baastrup
and Schou's riposte evoked a flurry of letters to the journal, published over the ensuing eight months. Experts in psychiatry and
the new drug treatments issued pronouncements for and against
lithium prophylaxis. Some focused on lithium's hazards.

Schou's reputation was at stake, and so was lithium's future.
Although Schou worked closely with Baastrup and others, he was
considered the foremost lithium expert and the major champion
of lithium as a prophylactic agent. As such he got much of the
credit—and blame—for the ongoing twists and turns in lithium's
standing. Was Schou a conscientious psychopharmacologist with a

groundbreaking treatment at hand, or was he a charlatan deluded by his irrational biases? Was lithium a minor accoutrement to the treatment of mania or a remarkable treatment advance? Seemingly levelheaded people weighed in on both sides.

Several of the letters to *The Lancet* supported Baastrup and Schou. Roy Hullin and his colleagues, writing from Yorkshire, said that they were in the midst of their own lithium prophylaxis study and getting similar results. Björn Laurell and Jan-Otto Ottosson, of Sweden, described their placebo-controlled prophylaxis study; it had started to show lithium's benefit, but they didn't complete the study because as they gained more experience with lithium they became convinced that lithium prevented relapses; patients were requesting lithium, and the researchers felt it was unethical to give patients placebo and deprive them of an effective treatment.

William Sargant, a prominent British psychiatrist known for the zeal with which he advocated physical treatments, including drugs—despite what many regarded as the absence of any solid evidence in support of them—dismissed Blackwell and Shepherd's methodological misgivings as trivial nitpicking. Underscoring his disdain for the contemporary research methods so dear to the Maudsley group, he wrote:

The article by Dr Blackwell and Professor Shepherd from the Maudsley Institute of Psychiatry, questioning statistically the value of lithium as a prophylactic in manic-depressive illness, calls for more comment. One must go on repeating the fact that if, in the past thirty years, one had ever paid very much attention to statistics, especially when they were not supported by clinical bedside findings, treatment progress in psychiatry in this country would not have got very far. . . . For the sake of England's present very high treatment reputation in world psychiatry let us try to keep a proper realization of the very limited value of crude statistics, especially when they are not confirmed by all the excellent clinical bedside work done in the past twenty or more years in this country. . . . And should we really . . . do more, probably valueless, double-blind sampling . . . with often such suffering and even suicide resulting from the control groups having to be kept on their inert tablets."[30]

Still, the foremost British psychiatrists endorsed Blackwell and Shepherd's views, and as a result, lithium was not welcome in the United Kingdom. The prevailing opinion in Britain was that there was simply no solid evidence to support the use of lithium as a prophylactic agent and precious little to recommend it as a treatment for mania. Aubrey Lewis, the eminent professor of psychiatry at the Maudsley, whose verdicts about psychiatric matters drew attention well beyond Britain's shores, described lithium treatment as "dangerous nonsense."[31]

Although the prophylaxis controversy centered on disagreements about research methods, it soon got personal—and nasty. Schou had made no secret of his brother's recurrent depressions, the presence of manic-depressive illness in other family members, and the fact that his brother and several others in his family had been successfully treated with lithium. Prompted, it seems, by this information, rumors circulated at the Maudsley that Schou himself was manic-depressive and on lithium. His critics hinted that this explained his enthusiasm for the drug, his seemingly unreasonable bias in favor of it, and his conviction that it was of value in the absence of a proper, controlled clinical trial.

When Schou heard about this sort of whispering, he unequivocally denied that he was either manic-depressive or taking lithium (and there was no evidence whatsoever that he was). Moreover, as Schou pointed out, these allegations were entirely beside the point. "I am not manic and never was in lithium treatment," he said. "But what difference would it make? Baastrup's and my data, arguments and conclusions are there for anyone to assess. Should data, arguments and conclusions presented by insane persons be disregarded rather than judged on their merits?"[32] Still, the ad hominem arguments persisted, and they hurt.

Reminiscing 40 years later, at age 86, Schou's dismay about Shepherd's derision seemed unabated:

> The term "enthusiastic advocate" has clung to me ever since Shepherd first used it. . . . I accept the first word . . . who would not be enthused when his or her research led to effective treatment of a long-lasting and serious illness? But the designation "advocate" I refuse to acknowledge. In the given context the term "advocate" can hardly have been meant as a compliment, an advocate being seen as a person who supports only one side of a case. A scientist, on the other hand, is someone who gathers all relevant evidence and then weighs it carefully before drawing a conclusion.[33]

Schou realized that without a conventional, controlled clinical trial, questions would remain about lithium's true worth. After considerable soul-searching, he and Baastrup decided that it was up to them to do that study. Blackwell, Shepherd, and other vociferous critics of lithium prophylaxis did not treat patients with lithium and showed no inclination to conduct their own investigation; further, Schou and Baastrup felt that they themselves were to some extent responsible for the uncertainty over lithium's prophylactic value and hence for the fact that some patients, particularly in the United Kingdom and United States, were being deprived of a potentially beneficial treatment. "If we had carried out our study with a double-blind design from the beginning," Schou said, "matters might have taken a different turn." In essence, "Baastrup and I felt deeply our obligation to the manic-depressive individuals around the world who were not given a chance with prophylactic lithium treatment. If the treatment was as good as our observations indicated, we were morally obliged to demonstrate this fact in such a way that psychiatrists everywhere would start using it."[34]

Still, Schou and Baastrup had grave misgivings about conducting a typical placebo-controlled trial where half the patients would get placebo rather than a drug that, in their minds, was highly beneficial, if not lifesaving: "Could we who were responsible for the patients' health, expose them to the risk of prolonged suffering or possibly suicide? Was consideration for the interests of manic-depressive patients in other hospitals or other countries sufficiently important to outweigh consideration for our own patients?"[35]

The extraordinary impact of lithium treatment on his younger brother's recurrent depressions—and on his quality of life—added to Schou's qualms. For 25 years, his brother had suffered severe depression every spring. "Then I started him on lithium," Schou said, "and the disease stopped. After years of being disabled he could resume work; he and his family were able to look to the future with new hope. Could Baastrup and I subject him or others like him to a . . . risk of being deprived of the treatment that had altered their lives so radically."[36]

In the end, Schou came up with a research design (double-blind discontinuation) that incorporated the stringent procedures of controlled research while minimizing the risks to patients. Eighty-four patients, all women and all treated at Glostrup Psychiatric Hospital, entered the study. Fifty had manic-depressive illness with episodes of both mania and depression (bipolar disorder), and 34 had recurrent depressions. All had been successfully treated with lithium for a year or more. For half of the patients, selected randomly, lithium capsules were replaced by identical placebos. The study was double-blind; neither the patients nor the psychiatrists treating and assessing them knew who was getting placebo and who lithium. When a patient relapsed, they were immediately provided suitable treatment. To expose as few patients as possible to placebo (and risk of relapse) and to get a definitive answer to the prophylaxis question as quickly as possible, the investigators used sequential analysis; they didn't wait for the end of the trial to analyze the results, as is usual; rather, they evaluated the data as they collected it, and they planned to stop the study as soon as it became clear that lithium-treated and placebo-treated patients differed significantly in number of relapses. They didn't have to wait long. After five months, 9 of the 34 patients with recurrent depression had relapsed. All had been on placebo; none of the 17 on lithium relapsed. In the group of 50 bipolar patients, 12 of the 22 on placebo had relapsed; none of the 28 on lithium had. So in five months, none of the patients treated with lithium had relapsed, whereas fully half on placebo had done so. Lithium's prophylactic effect was undeniable.

Schou and his collaborators sent the paper reporting these results to *The Lancet*. Its editor rejected it, feeling that "lithium had received enough publicity." This affront, added to the others from the Brits, was maddening. Schou believed it was only fair that *The Lancet* publish his paper, since it was largely a response to the Blackwell and Shepherd critique that had appeared in its pages. At a psychopharmacology meeting in the Caribbean, Schou let W. Linford Rees, a prominent British psychiatrist, know of his exasperation with *The Lancet*. Upon returning to England, Rees intervened with *The Lancet*'s editor on behalf of Baàstrup and Schou, pointing out the importance of their study. The journal then agreed to publish it, and it appeared in the August 15, 1970, issue.[37]

The double-blind discontinuation study effectively settled the prophylaxis issue. John Cade, who, after his 1949 study, did no lithium research himself, had nevertheless kept up with the ensuing research and particularly with the work of Mogens Schou. They had corresponded since the early 1960s and visited each other several times in the 1970s. Cade was well aware of the dispute about prophylaxis and its acrimony. When the double-blind discontinuation article appeared, Cade was delighted. In a letter to Schou, he thanked him for "the copy of your memorable paper that was published (so reluctantly) by the *Lancet*." Cade went on to express what many in Schou's camp must have felt: "They did not have the decency to produce an editorial annotation acknowledging that you and Poul had K-Oed Blackwell and Shepherd in the final round! No matter. Your contention has been proven so conclusively that the whole world must be persuaded."[38]

And so it was. Doubts about lithium's importance were almost entirely put to rest. Several rigorously controlled studies over the next few years from England, the United States, and elsewhere confirmed lithium's prophylactic value. Those studies—along with dozens of "open" investigations from the late 1960s onward and the buildup of affirming clinical experience—established lithium as a uniquely effective prophylactic agent. It didn't work in all patients, but it prevented bouts of illness in the majority of those with both recurring depressions and repeated episodes of both mania and depression. Alone among the agents introduced 60 years ago in the first wave of psychiatric drugs, lithium is still widely used and remains the gold standard for the treatment of manic-depressive illness.

Some historians of psychiatry have suggested that Cade's discovery would have been forgotten without Schou's persistent and systematic research. Cade himself acknowledged Schou as "the person who has done most" to gain recognition for lithium "by validating and extending my original observations." Schou, for his part, never failed to point out that Cade's lithium observations provided the inspiration for his research, and he invariably spoke and wrote admiringly about Cade's lithium research and his personal qualities.

It took Schou and his collaborators two decades to get lithium accepted worldwide. Along the way, Schou was vilified and his scientific integrity questioned. Finally, though, the accolades started coming. In 1974, for their work with lithium, Cade and Schou shared the International Kittay Scientific Foundation Award. Over the following decades, Schou received several honorary doctorates and numerous research awards. He was nominated at least twice for a Nobel Prize. In 1987, he got a Lasker Award, often referred to as America's Nobel, for lithium treatment of manic-depressive illness. Although he appreciated these accolades, as he said upon receiving one of these awards: "For me every single patient whose life was changed radically by lithium outweighs honors and awards. I trust that you understand and agree."[39]

The controversy between Schou and Blackwell and Shepherd over lithium prophylaxis—and the acrimony it generated—was never fully laid to rest. Blackwell, who played rugby at the highest competitive level (at one point, he captained the formidable Guy's Rugby Football Club), didn't give up easily. Turning his attention to the discontinuation study, he wrote several pieces in the early 1970s criticizing its methods and conclusions. By 1980, though, he had accepted (sort of) the consensus regarding lithium's utility. In that year, he said: "I believe that we were right to make the methodologic points that we did and that they were (and remain) valid. We were also wrong. I think that the weight of clinical conviction by this date is convincing and that lithium has a place in the prevention of manic relapses."[40] Still, Blackwell never completely renounced his skepticism: "However, I also think that the whole area of prophylaxis and maintenance therapy should be very closely examined. . . . I suspect that what has changed is not the weight of *scientific* evidence so much as the sheer *clinical* consensus concerning efficacy. If one were to submit current data to equally rigorous scrutiny it might still fall short of 'proof.'"[41]

Shepherd was another matter. He never commented publicly on Baastrup and Schou's definitive discontinuation study, and his truculence did not go unnoticed. Jules Angst, an expert on the course of manic-depressive illness and a founder of the International Group for the Study of Affective Disorders (IGSAD), a forum for leading researchers to exchange information and discuss their findings, had asked Shepherd to join the group. Schou first presented the positive results of the discontinuation study at an IGSAD meeting. "Michael Shepherd remained silent during the discussion," Angst said, "and when asked for his opinion replied 'no comment.' At the end of that year I asked him to retire from the group. After his refusal to discuss Mogens Schou's presentation I felt his continued membership was inappropriate."[42]

For the rest of his life (he died in 1995), Shepherd maintained in interviews and in his lectures and writings that the claims for lithium prophylaxis were exaggerated, unjustified, and unproven. At best, as he said at a conference in 1973, "lithium should be regarded as a substance with exciting possibilities for scientific enquiry."[43]

Years later, after the prophylaxis storm had somewhat dissipated, Erik Strömgren asked Shepherd, whom he knew well, why he had continued this "unreasonable" and "denigrating" controversy. According to Strömgren, Shepherd "quite openly" explained that the attacks were "simply due to the fact that English psychiatry under the reign of Aubrey Lewis did not distinguish between psychogenic and endogenous depression [depression caused by stress, as opposed to the sort that is part of manic-depressive illness], and if lithium were to be recommended against depression, all doctors in England would use it against all types of depression with the result that many patients not in need of it would only suffer damage from it—therefore lithium must be ravaged with fire and sword."[44]

Nonetheless, the evidence supporting lithium's value was too compelling to ignore, and psychiatrists in the United Kingdom took it on. Skeptics periodically came forward—the British psychiatrist Joanna Moncrieff, a vociferous opponent of psychiatric drug treatment in general, wrote articles in the mid-1990s calling into question lithium's usefulness for anything—but the weight of clinical opinion supported lithium's importance. By the mid-1970s, those most determined to vanquish lithium had left the scene: Aubrey Lewis, who had proclaimed that lithium was "dangerous nonsense," retired in 1966 and died in 1975; Michael Shepherd left psychopharmacology in 1967 to pursue an illustrious career in psychiatric epidemiology; and Barry Blackwell emigrated to the United States in 1968 to work for a drug company.

Schou investigated lithium and wrote and spoke about it until his death in 2005. He tackled everything from the impact of lithium on artistic productivity to its effect on the kidney, from its safety in pregnancy to strategies for avoiding toxicity. When other drugs that seemed to have some prophylactic benefit came along, Schou identified the kinds of patients most likely to benefit from them and the sorts of patients who did particularly well on lithium. Because lithium had no commercial support, Schou took it upon himself to collect and disseminate the available information. In addition to his steady outpouring of research reports and scholarly reviews, he wrote several nontechnical books about lithium for patients and their families.

Schou died on September 29, 2005, at age 86, just days after returning from a meeting in Poland of the International Group for the Study of Lithium-Treated Patients. He collapsed while he was working on a manuscript and succumbed to pneumonia a few hours later. Over the decades, he aided an untold number of manic-depressive sufferers. Convinced that lithium was an important treatment, he never stopped conducting research related to it; and until his death in 2005, he strove to educate both professionals and the lay public about its value.

EPILOGUE

AFTER HIS 1949 landmark study, Cade did no further research with lithium. From today's perspective, this is somewhat perplexing. Given the intense competition among present-day scientists for research grants and publication in prestigious journals, it is inconceivable that someone making a discovery like Cade's would simply drop it, leaving it to others to pursue. Part of Cade's disinclination to do further lithium research probably stemmed from his worry about lithium toxicity. But that's not the whole story.

Cade's son Jack speculated about his father's seeming indifference to conducting further lithium research: "In those days, in the late 1940s, when one published a paper, people didn't go on to keep publishing as they do now . . . he was a busy clinician and administrator . . . I don't think he felt the need to be at the front. He felt he had done what he could and left the rest to others with more research skills, to follow this up. He also moved on to other areas. He was always curious about what caused schizophrenia."[1]

And Cade himself, in a letter to Neil Johnson in August 1980, commented on his attitude toward his lithium discovery: "Oddly enough, I did not frantically pursue it. I knew the results were valid and simply cast my bread upon the waters. It was, I now realize, perilous to do this. Fortunately it was turned into cake, preeminently by Schou and his coworkers."[2]

But encouraged by his success with lithium, Cade did proceed to investigate a number of similar elements to see if they had psychological effects: "It was inevitable, having thus been unexpectedly presented with a therapeutic magic wand, that one would plunge one's hand time and again into the same lucky dip."[3]

He found that salts of rubidium and caesium, alkali metals very similar to lithium and close neighbors on the periodic table, had no effects in guinea pigs or rats. Cade looked into salts of cerium, a rare-earth element. When he injected them into rats, they became sedated, as they did when injected with similar rare-earth elements. But Cade found that oral doses of cerium carbonate had no discernible effect on him or on four psychotic patients.

Still, Cade's travels through the periodic table did not leave him totally empty-handed. He took a look at strontium, another alkaline metal, and he had a rather complex rationale for doing so. ("It was not simply that I was working my way systematically through the periodic table.") He had shown that people with severe depression and schizophrenia seem to differ from healthy people in the way they metabolize magnesium, an element that plays a critical role in cell chemistry and brain cell excitability. Since strontium is very similar to magnesium, Cade thought that strontium might modify the abnormal magnesium metabolism. Further, strontium salts had been widely used in medicine and did not seem to have toxic effects.

Once again, Cade himself was the guinea pig. When he found that strontium carbonate in a single dose up to 4 mg did not upset his stomach or otherwise make him ill, he proceeded to take 4 mg three times a day for five days. Cade noted a tranquilizing effect: "I am not a tension-prone individual, but I was under considerable irritating stress that week and was surprised by my equanimity under the circumstances."[4] By the fifth day, he was quite drowsy.

After stopping the strontium, he slept for most of a day but otherwise suffered no ill effects.

Over the next ten months, Cade gave strontium to 30 patients with a variety of psychiatric problems. None of the patients with chronic schizophrenia or serious depression improved, but 2 patients with severe anxiety were completely better in two days, and after about a week on strontium a few with acute schizophrenia and 2 of the 3 patients with mania got substantially better. (Cade allowed that this improvement could have been a result of spontaneous remission.) Many of the patients whose chief mental symptoms did not improve became less restless and sometimes drowsy.

Rats and guinea pigs injected with strontium in doses comparable to the ones given to humans became sedated, "confirming the validity of the tranquilizing effect observed in man." Cade believed he was onto something. Summing up his research with strontium, he said, "There is no doubt whatever that it is substantially anxiolytic, safe, effective and cheap. . . . Strontium may also prove to have . . . value for research in this field."[5]

Cade never formally published his strontium research in a scientific journal, but he spoke about it. When he was invited to talk about his lithium discovery at an April 1970 symposium on "Discoveries in Biological Psychiatry," he concluded his lecture, titled "The Story of Lithium," with a detailed description of his strontium work. Cade's lecture, including his comments about strontium, appeared in the proceedings of the symposium.[6]

Later that year, at Mogens Schou's invitation, Cade gave a lecture in Risskov. Schou had asked Cade to speak about lithium, and Cade had replied that he'd be "delighted" to do so. But things didn't work out that way: "I had exhorted him to give an account of the background for his discovery of lithium's antimanic effect," Schou said, "however, against all expectations he spoke about his investigations with strontium."[7] Cade's claim that strontium had promise as a psychiatric treatment and, at the very least, was "worthy of further study" failed to grip his colleagues (Cade's data were not particularly compelling), and strontium as a psychiatric treatment never got off the ground. Today, strontium compounds are used, as they were in Cade's day, for the treatment of bone disease.

In 1950, probably because of his lithium research, Cade was promoted to medical superintendent at Bundoora Hospital; and in 1951, again probably because of his research activities, he was invited to give the prestigious Beattie-Smith Lectures, annual public lectures about psychiatry presented at the University of Melbourne. In 1952, continuing on this quite rapid upward trajectory, Cade was appointed superintendent of Melbourne's esteemed Royal Park Psychiatric Hospital and dean of its Clinical School. Cade remained at Royal Park until his retirement in 1977.

Despite his administrative, teaching, and clinical responsibilities, Cade continued to come up with, and test, hypotheses about the causes of the major psychiatric illnesses—schizophrenia and manic depression. Convinced that these disorders involved a disturbance in brain chemistry—in part because of lithium's profound impact on mania—Cade looked for abnormalities in the chemicals that brain cells depend on: sodium, potassium, and magnesium among them. Through the 1960s, he did a series of studies in seriously ill psychiatric patients, examining the plasma levels of these chemicals. For the most part, he found slight, if any, deviations from normal levels. But it didn't take much in the way of actual data to persuade Cade that he was on the right track. Discussing a plasma level study that showed a possible abnormality in the way some depressed patients metabolize magnesium, he said, "It is clear that another highly significant biochemical correlate of melancholia has been identified."[8] Cade's biochemical studies were largely disregarded. We now know, in fact, that plasma levels of these chemicals are not a reliable measure of brain chemistry.

It seems that Cade's brain never stopped simmering. His talent for educated speculation, for weaving disparate facts into more or less plausible hypotheses, was a particular strength; it far outweighed the sophistication of his research methods or his interest in and aptitude for subjecting a hypothesis to a rigorous test. Schou, who admired Cade and became very fond of him, characterized him as an artistic scientist as opposed to a systematic one. The systematic scientist, Schou said, fits the popular image of a scientist. He works methodically, "going forward step by step. He starts at point A and proceeds via points B and C to reach point D." The artistic scientist, on the other hand, "works by intuition as well as by logic. Starting at point A he also proceeds to point D, but not necessarily via B and C; eventually he may even arrive at points E or F. How he does so is not always clear but he does it."[9]

Schou counted himself among the systematic types. But he emphasized that both artistic and systematic scientists are essential for scientific progress. "The systematic scientist," he said, "may add to our knowledge with solidity and precision, but the artistic scientist is often the real innovator, because he has the livelier phantasy and perhaps the greater courage."

Cade's penchant for informed speculation, for inductive leaps— indeed, for fantasy—allowed him to make his lithium discovery. But it is the rare scientist, however systematic, artistic, or courageous, who makes even one discovery of that import; more than one is simply too much to expect. So although after 1949 Cade was never short of ideas—some more plausible than others—neither those ideas nor his later research left a mark.

Still, the fertility of his imagination is notable. Postulating that the geographical distribution of schizophrenia might shed some light on its cause, Cade carried out a survey examining the incidence of hospital admissions for schizophrenia in the different urban and rural areas of Victoria. He noted that areas with a low incidence of schizophrenia had a relative abundance of fruit trees, especially stone fruit trees, such as peach, apricot, and plum. Cade hypothesized that fruit contains a "protective factor" that when deficient allows schizophrenia to develop.[10]

Two years later, in a speculative tour de force, he hypothesized that mongolism (now called Down syndrome) results from inadequate manganese in the diet of pregnant women. He conveyed this hypothesis in a letter to the *Medical Journal of Australia* and described how he got to it: chondrodystrophy (abnormal cartilage and bone development) in chick embryos bears some similarity, Cade believed, to Down syndrome; chondrodystrophy results from manganese deficiency in the hen's diet; tea is an important dietary source of manganese; and, according to his obstetrician colleagues, Cade said, many pregnant women stop drinking tea. So Down syndrome, he speculated, may result from manganese deficiency.[11] Cade thought it might be worthwhile to test this hypothesis by encouraging pregnant women to drink tea to see if that influenced the incidence of Down syndrome. The pregnant women of Australia were saved from this fate when in 1959, one year after Cade's letter appeared, French researchers traced the cause of Down syndrome to an extra chromosome.

In the decades following 1949, Cade was busy with other matters as well. He was devoted to Jean and, unlike his own father, was an involved and loving dad. He had four sons; Jack and David born before he went to war, Peter born in 1948, and Richard in 1950. Jack, David, and Richard became physicians; Peter became a science technologist. They all have children of their own—14 in total at last count.

A daughter, Mary, was born in 1947. She lived for only one day. Cade had a lasting memory of carrying his daughter's tiny coffin in one hand at her small funeral. Family members consider Mary's death the greatest tragedy in Cade's life.

Cade became one of Australia's foremost teachers of psychiatry. University of Melbourne medical students came to Royal Park on Saturday mornings to hear his lectures. Bernard Carroll, an eminent psychiatrist known for his work in biological psychiatry, was one of those students:

John Cade would teach us psychopathology and his style was very Kraeplinian. He was up on stage with two chairs, one for the patient and one for him. An assistant would be hovering around and the patients would be lined up off stage. He would signal to stage right for a patient to be brought in and would say, in a very Edwardian authoritarian manner, 'Ladies and gentlemen, I'm now going to demonstrate a patient with schizophrenia'. The patient would be brought and John Cade would put the schizophrenic patient through his hoops, send the patient off stage left, signal again to stage right and say, 'Ladies and gentlemen I'm now going to demonstrate a patient with mania so you should pay close attention to the differences between them.' His style was very autocratic and old fashioned, but in many ways effective.[12]

In 1970, describing his lithium research to a newspaper reporter, Cade noted that he had worked by himself—and preferred it that way. "I've always been a lone wolf," he said. "I'd be absolutely useless as head of a team, I'm sure."[13] But as much as working alone and independently may have served his lithium discovery, Cade was hardly a "lone wolf" in his other professional roles. In addition to the administrative obligations that came with being a dean and hospital superintendent, Cade took an active role in psychiatric organizations and did so from the start of his psychiatric career. In 1939, just before the outbreak of war, he was among the mental hospital psychiatrists who formed a group called the Mental Hygiene Medical Officers Association (MHMOA). Among other things, it advocated research in mental hospitals and public education about the new treatments available in the mental hospitals.

In 1946, Cade was a founding member of the Australasian Association of Psychiatrists, and when in 1964 the Royal Australian and New Zealand College of Psychiatrists (RANZCP) replaced the association, Cade was among the select few who were elected foundation fellows. Five years later, he was its president.

Cade had an encyclopedic knowledge of psychiatry and was thoroughly conversant about both its history and the treatments and theories of his time. But he had his biases, and one of them was psychoanalysis. It seemed that he just couldn't stand it, and his objections seemed to rest on both moral and scientific grounds. In his 1951 Beattie-Smith Lecture, he let loose:

The decadent Vienna of the last years of the Austro-Hungarian Empire warped more minds than Schikelgruber's [Hitler's]). I believe that Freudian psychology has cast a blight upon the minds of men that will last perhaps another fifty years. . . . The really great error that appals me is Freud's implicit assumption of psychic determinism, the criminal's best friend for a generation. The argument has been, roughly: "Poor fellow, he couldn't help himself; he was an automaton in the grip of that ravening demon, his unconscious" . . . this denial of free will and hence of criminal responsibility has discredited us perhaps more than any other assertion we may make.[14]

Cade's objections to psychoanalysis did not arise from a failure to comprehend it. He had read Freud's work extensively and had a sophisticated understanding of psychoanalytic theory; he just didn't buy it: "Freud's theories of pan-sexualism and psycho-sexual development are to many, including myself, simply not true. The Freudian reply is, of course, that this is because such ideas are repugnant to me and I am therefore psychoresistive to their acceptance. Well, I am certainly resistive to accepting anything for which I cannot see sufficient evidence."[15]

The plain-speaking, self-deprecating Cade, who had a way with words and, in particular, a flair for the unpretentious turn of a phrase, found the abstruseness of psychoanalytic terminology irritating and offensive: "Let me utter a word of plaintive protest concerning the esoteric jargon which has grown up as part of this fascinating phantasmagoria. . . . I saw psychoanalysis defined as the art of describing the commonplace in terms of the incomprehensible."[16]

Cade was not alone in his skepticism. Still, in the mid-twentieth century, psychoanalysis dominated psychiatric thinking in Australia as it did elsewhere, especially among psychiatrists who taught in universities and treated patients in private practice. As Cade said, for many psychiatrists, "Freud is a very great god indeed." And the psychiatrists who embraced psychoanalysis made up an influential segment of the Australian psychiatric community. Cade's vociferous objections to psychoanalysis and his insistence on biological explanations for mental illness diverged from mainstream thinking, and in many quarters they got a frosty reception. But they were welcomed by a number of psychiatrists, particularly Catholic ones, and by the Catholic Church. For the Church, Cade's ideas were a refreshing antidote to the godless and altogether repugnant psychoanalytic concepts. The Church found in Cade an agreeable voice for psychiatry. It called upon him to lecture about psychiatry and mental health to trainee priests and other audiences.

Cade was a devout Catholic, and he took on the role of Church spokesperson on psychiatric matters. In addition to lecturing on the Church's behalf, Cade wrote a column about mental health for *The Messenger*, a Jesuit magazine that went to thousands of Australian Catholics. He wrote under the pseudonym Mensana (from the Latin for "a healthy mind"), and he proffered advice on everything from child-rearing to insomnia. Most of his columns provided solid, practical information. In January 1952, he addressed a column to the sleepless. His suggestion for bringing on slumber was eminently sensible and is a staple of today's sleep experts: "Relax brother—take it easy. Start from your eyes and work downwards relaxing each group of muscles in turn."[17] But occasionally his prejudices came to the fore. In his December 1951 column, "Bringing up Children," he gave vent to one of his favorite peeves: "I'd sooner a child were brought up by good Catholic parents, who had not read one paragraph in press or magazines on how to bring up their children than by the most learned psychiatrist whose approach was governed solely by the findings of modern secular psychology."[18]

Cade's objections to "modern secular psychology" became well known. But his rejection of psychoanalytic thinking was more nuanced than it sometimes appeared. He never backed off from his conviction that psychoanalysis and other psychological theories are useless when it comes to understanding and treating the major psychiatric disorders—schizophrenia and manic depression. But Cade made it clear that the detailed exploration of a patient's development that takes place in psychoanalysis has an important place in the care of people with troubled relationships, neurotic disturbances, and so-called personality disorders. Indeed, in *Mending the Mind*, Cade's brief history of psychiatry published in 1979, the year before he died, Cade acknowledged: "Freud has made a major contribution to the care of troubled minds, if not sick ones in the medical sense. He has shown how necessary it is to spend endless hours painstakingly attempting to discover how the personality evolves . . . to reveal what are the dynamics, the moulding influences, and how the person was shaped by them and is still reacting to them."[19]

Notwithstanding his declarations to the contrary, Cade was hardly immune to the powerful ideas about the mind that had captured so many of his colleagues. Even his Mensana columns were touched by psychoanalytic concepts. In a column about obsessions and scrupulosity, Cade wrote: "The worry and indecision engendered by unresolved guilt extends to all sorts of unrelated thoughts and actions. We may become over-scrupulous about other things as a compensation for being under-scrupulous about something else. It is possible that the original incident was in the distant past and practically forgotten although the attitude of mind it generated then has persisted in some degree and coloured our life ever since."[20] Although Cade does not mention Freud or psychoanalysis here, he alludes to the unconscious, repression, and displacement, ideas straight from the psychoanalytic playbook.

In 1955, the Democratic Labor Party (DLP) came into being as a result of a split in the Australian Labor Party. The DLP was supported by the Catholic Church, and most of its members were Catholic. It was stridently anticommunist and socially conservative, opposing abortion, homosexuality, and other sorts of "permissiveness." Cade was, in some ways, a good fit for the DLP. His anti-Freud pronouncements were compatible with the DLP's policies. He became their go-to psychiatrist.

Yet Cade never fit completely into one ideological box. Devout though he was, he could veer from Catholic doctrine when he believed that common sense or science trumped it. In 1972, he gave an address to the Annual Congress of the Australian and New Zealand College of Psychiatrists titled "Masturbational Madness: An Historical Annotation." With unrestrained irony, Cade set forth the late nineteenth- and early twentieth-century warnings about the dangers of masturbation, which included, among many other things, mental illness: "It is salutary in this amoral and licentious age," he said, "to again draw attention to the disastrous consequences of the evil habit that destroyed Onan. . . . Far too little has been written in recent years about the vice named after him: far too few warnings given. A spirit of skepticism regarding the tragic consequences of this unnatural and disgusting practice has become wide-spread even amongst otherwise sensible and intelligent members of our profession. . . . For the benefit of the innumerable young people at risk, the trend must be neutralized. They must be made to realize the perils of perversity."[21] Cade went on to entertain his audience with the solemn pronouncements of an early twentieth-century physician on the dire consequences of masturbation, including insanity. His irony offered no comfort to traditional Church doctrine on the matter.

In 1973, Cade contributed a paper titled "An Eclectic Psychiatrist Looks at Homosexuality" to a symposium on liberation movements and psychiatry. The younger colleague who organized the symposium and invited him expected that "he would express a strong view that homosexuality was a psychiatric disorder requiring treatment." But to his surprise, Cade's views were "remarkably liberal." Cade was clear on both his personal and professional positions: "I am an elderly heterosexual happily married grandfather and being a Catholic accept insofar as my own personal life is concerned Catholic teaching in the field of sexual morality—but I hasten to add that as a doctor I regard it as highly irrelevant and always mischievous to make moral judgments on patients' problems and attitudes."[22]

As for whether or not homosexuality is "psychiatrically abnormal," a matter that his colleagues had yet to agree on, Cade was clear: "My own view is that a stable homosexual relationship is certainly not more psychiatrically abnormal than nail biting, or thumb sucking or doodling or cigarette smoking. If homosexuality is perverse and an illness or abnormality surely deliberately inhaling large quantities of filthy disease producing smoke into one's lungs day after day should also be defined in similar terms."[23] (Cade was an inveterate smoker.)

IN 1963, Schou wrote to Cade telling him of his work with lithium. Over the next 15 years, they corresponded regularly and visited each other twice. On more than one occasion, they expressed both privately and publicly their gratitude to each other for, on the one hand, introducing lithium treatment, and, on the other, nurturing its development. In 1970, Schou introduced Cade to an audience gathered in Risskov to hear Cade speak, describing him as the man who "introduced lithium into psychiatry and described its antimanic effect." Schou continued: "I do not have it in my power to endow knighthoods or honorary degrees but permit me to express quite simply to you, John Cade, the gratitude of all the psychiatrists and scientists for whom your work has been an inspiration and a stimulus. I think also I may thank you on behalf of the very, very many patients all over the world who have, and the still many more who will, derive benefit from and have their lives entirely changed through treatment with the drug you introduced."[24]

On the same occasion, Cade said (referring to Schou's lithium work): "I feel rather like a woman who as a girl had an illegitimate child and had it adopted out. And now, 20 years later, I am visiting the adoptive parents and finding out what a big fine boy he has grown into, but knowing far less about him than his adoptive parents."[25]

Throughout the 1950s, it became increasingly clear that with careful attention to side effects and measurement of serum levels, lithium therapy was safe. Cade stopped prohibiting its use, and by 1957, doctors at Royal Park were prescribing it. Although Cade did no further research with lithium, starting in 1967 he wrote several articles and book chapters about it, recounting the "story" of his discovery and providing reviews and updates on how lithium should be applied. On several occasions, he proposed that in addition to its acknowledged value in the treatment of mania, lithium could be useful in the treatment of some patients with schizophrenia, particularly those who show symptoms of mania.

When, by the late 1960s, lithium therapy became widely used, Cade was credited with its discovery, and the accolades started coming. In April 1970, he was among the illustrious psychiatric researchers who received the Taylor Manor Hospital Award for their groundbreaking drug treatment discoveries. Cade and the other researchers recounted the stories of their breakthroughs at a symposium on "Discoveries in Biological Psychiatry," held in Baltimore. That year the American Psychiatric Association named him a Distinguished Fellow. In 1974, for their lithium discovery, Cade and Schou shared the $25,000 Kittay Scientific Foundation Award. Bestowed in New York, it was at that time the world's foremost and largest psychiatric prize. Reserved, unpretentious, and self-deprecating though he was, Cade fully enjoyed these tributes.

In 1976, he was made an Officer of the Order of Australia, one of the first to receive that honor. It was only in the previous year that Queen Elizabeth II had announced the scrapping of the knighthood and other British honors for citizens of Australia and their replacement by the Order of Australia. Noting that Cade "was not entirely immune to . . . social approbation," Neil Johnson recalled Cade's consternation at perhaps having just missed a knighthood: "John confessed to me that he would have much preferred to be known as *Sir* John Cade, than the rather dull (as it seemed to him) AO. To have missed out on a knighthood by little more than a year struck him as being hard luck of the worst kind. 'Anyway', he said to me, 'it sounds as though someone's saying 'John Cade, eh? Oh!'."[26]

The recognition continued. In 1977, he was the guest of honor and guest speaker at the First British Lithium Congress, held at the

University of Lancaster, and in 1978, he was the guest of honor at the International Lithium Conference in New York City. In 1979, the Collegium Internationale Neuro-Psychopharmacologicum (CINP) made him an honorary member.

Cade retired from Royal Park in January 1977. He and Jean moved to a Cade family home in Toorak, an affluent suburb of Melbourne. Among other things, retirement allowed Cade frequent visits to the zoo with his grandchildren. But he did not fully sever his ties to medicine and psychiatry. Cade served as chair of the RANZCP's Victorian Branch until his death in 1980 and on the Medical Board of Victoria (he had been appointed to the board in 1970 and remained on it until his death).

Moreover, after leaving Royal Park, Cade wrote his brief (108-page) history of twentieth-century psychiatry, titled *Mending the Mind*. Meant for the layperson, it came out in 1979. On the cover is a cartoon showing a psychiatrist lifting the top of a patient's skull and peering at his brain. The book goes on from there—pungent, witty, forthright, and packed with personal and entertaining asides. In introducing the chapter about anxiety, Cade wrote:

> No man . . . has ever been totally and permanently free from anxiety. It is an inseparable part of human existence and man since the beginning of time has always sought means to assuage it. He has propitiated the gods, he has ingested tranquilliz-ers. . . . He has found marvelous herbs and potions includ-ing fungi, roots, leaves, flowers fruits, and gases. . . . He has sought the support of his fellows, individually and collectively. He has hastened for counsel and support from wise men, sages, yogis, prophets. He has looked to the interpretation of his dreams. He has been persuaded to be relieved of his anxiety on the instalment plan or by deconditioning, in which he starts by facing a little fear and works up to confront a big one.[27]

More than one colleague found it remarkable that in his chapter on lithium, Cade recounts the discovery of lithium treatment, including the guinea pig experiments and the first trial in patients, without once mentioning that he was the one who did it. Likewise, he describes the detection of vitamin deficiencies among mental hospital patients as the work of a "young medical officer," without mentioning that he was the medical officer.

Cade had been an inveterate smoker all his adult life; despite his family's pleas, he never stopped. His son Jack believes that his smoking habit became "irrevocably entrenched" during his incarceration at Changi. Incorrigible though he was, Cade was not by any definition a heavy smoker. In a highly routinized way he smoked seven cigarettes a day, one each at breakfast, morning tea, lunch, afternoon tea, and dinner and two in the evening. Nonetheless, even light smoking drastically increases the risk of several cancers, among them cancer of the esophagus.

In early September 1980, Cade had some trouble swallowing. Within a week he was diagnosed with cancer of the esophagus. Surgery turned out to be untenable; on opening him up, the surgeon found him riddled with cancer. Chemotherapy followed, leaving him weak and ill. As death came close, Cade told Jack that he wished to be buried near his parents at Yan Yean, a rural suburb of Melbourne, in the "simplest box." He died at age 68, at St Vincent's Hospital on November 16, 1980.

Cade's death in 1980 brought a slew of memorial tributes. Shortly after he died, Royal Park named its adult acute ward the John Cade Unit. In 1982, at the CINP conference in Jerusalem, Mogens Schou delivered the first John Cade Memorial Lecture. And that year the Victorian Branch of the RANZCP established the John Cade Memorial Medal, awarded each year to Victorian medical students in their final year who place first in their school's psychiatry examinations. In 1983, the faculty of medicine at the University of Melbourne introduced the John Cade Memorial Prize.

As of the writing of this book, John Cade is not a household name in Australia or anywhere else. But to psychiatrists throughout the world familiar at all with the history of psychiatric drugs, he is an iconic figure. For Australian psychiatrists he holds singular importance. Seventy years after his lithium discovery, he remains Australia's preeminent psychiatrist. When in 2013 Australia's National Health and Medical Research Council offered a generously funded five-year fellowship for mental health research, they named it the NHMRC John Cade Fellowship in Mental Health Research.

THE SIMPLE salt that John Cade put to such good use remains alive and well. The raft of other psychiatric drugs—antidepressants, antipsychotics, and antianxiety agents—discovered in the decade after lithium came on the scene and which, along with lithium, launched the "psychopharmacologic revolution" are little used today. They have been largely replaced by somewhat better variants. Lithium, alone among these pioneering treatments, continues to be widely used. It is, in fact, still the gold standard treatment for manic-depressive illness. Despite the introduction of several new agents for the long-term treatment of manic depression, lithium remains unsurpassed in its ability to prevent attacks of mania and depression. Over the past 50 years, it has provided a normal life for millions of people with manic-depressive illness. In doing so, it has—incidentally—saved billions of dollars in health care costs.[28]

Needless to say, lithium is not perfect; about 30 percent of manic-depressive people don't benefit from it, and it has some troublesome side effects. As we have discussed elsewhere in this book, the lithium dose required for treatment and the dose that produces dangerous toxicity are close. So, people can get quite sick if they inadvertently take too much lithium or if their body's ability to eliminate lithium changes. As long as serum lithium levels are watched and the levels are kept within the proper range, toxicity is readily avoided.

Lithium can disturb the activity of the thyroid gland, and most troublesome, it can hinder kidney function. Unchecked, the disturbance in kidney function can progress, in a small number of people, to kidney damage. Serious thyroid and kidney problems are unlikely to occur when the treating doctor carries out blood tests to evaluate the state of these organs on a regular basis.

Although it is abundantly clear that lithium has transformed the treatment of manic-depressive illness and enhanced (and saved) the lives of millions, it's difficult to come up with an accurate estimate of how many people are taking lithium today. Not all countries track prescriptions, and there is no incentive for the pharmaceutical industry to keep a tally of those who use it. Based on the prevalence of manic-depressive illness and the probable fraction of its victims who get lithium, a conservative guess would be that 1 to 2 out of every 1,000 people in industrialized countries are now on lithium. Accordingly, at least 250,000 U.S. adults are taking lithium.

Although lithium is the best treatment for preventing manic and depressive episodes—certainly it is the treatment that has the most evidence behind it—not everyone who could benefit from lithium gets it. Prescribing patterns vary from country to country. In some European and Scandinavian countries, about 50 percent of people with manic-depressive illness take lithium; far fewer patients in the United States (about 10 percent) take it.[29] A major reason for the underuse of lithium in the United States is the introduction and marketing of valproate. In the mid-1980s, valproate, an anticonvulsant widely used for preventing seizures, started to gain attention as a treatment for mania and as a prophylactic agent, or mood stabilizer, in manic-depressive illness. In 1995, the FDA approved valproate as a treatment for mania, and Abbott, the drug company making it, began to promote it aggressively. Clinical trials showed that valproate could both alleviate mania and prevent manic and depressive episodes. It had no advantages over lithium in this regard and for the most part was less effective than lithium. But the combination of hard-hitting marketing and the impression that valproate was safer than lithium and easier to use (it didn't require blood level measurements or attention to kidney and thyroid performance) turned the tide in its favor. So valproate, despite troublesome side effects of its own, including a significant incidence of fetal abnormalities, became more widely used in the United States than lithium and has remained so.

Experts agree that lithium is now used far less than it should be—certainly in the United States. There is a growing concern that given the lack of drug company support for lithium, the constant introduction of new vigorously promoted competing (but less effective) agents, and the common perception that lithium is tricky to use and dangerous, the latest generation of psychiatrists are simply not learning how to use it.

Nonetheless, a lithium renaissance may be in the making. Recent books and scholarly reviews devoted to contemporary lithium research affirm its unique value in stopping attacks of mania and depression. Lithium provides benefit to people with all varieties of manic-depressive illness: the classic type (periodic bouts of both mania and depression), now called bipolar I disorder; bouts of depression interspersed with hypomania (periods of exuberance less severe than mania), so-called bipolar II disorder; and, recurrent episodes of depression alone.

Although lithium can put a stop to the recurrent mood swings for many if not most of the patients with these conditions, its effects appear to be most predictable and robust in people with a classic manic-depressive illness. This "classic" form of the illness usually begins in early adulthood. Periodic attacks of deep, agonizing depression alternate with bouts of mania characterized by euphoria, intense excitement, bizarre thinking, and irrational behavior. These episodes of mood (technically known as affective) disturbance occur up to three times a year and last for months. Between these episodes, the victims are quite well—calm, clearheaded, and essentially indistinguishable from their healthy counterparts. But inevitably, without treatment, all hell once again breaks loose. This form of manic-depressive illness (as opposed to varieties where the attacks of affective disturbance involve irritability or a mixture of moods, the episodes occur more frequently, or the interludes between episodes are less trouble-free) is so remarkably and reliably modified by lithium that one expert suggested that it be called Cade's disease.

Fueling the continued interest in and allegiance to lithium treatment has been the growing recognition over the past few decades that lithium therapy alone among treatments for manic-depressive illness brings about a striking reduction in suicide. People with manic-depressive illness are unusually likely to kill themselves. About 6 percent die by suicide, a rate of suicide 10 to 20 times higher than that of the general population.[30] Over the past several decades, dozens of studies, some controlled clinical trials and other more naturalistic investigations of suicide risk before and after lithium treatment, have shown that lithium treatment produces a notable decrease in suicide—about a 10-fold reduction.

Other drugs used in the long-term treatment of manic-depressive illness, including antidepressants, valproate, and other anticonvulsants, do not seem to have this anti-suicide effect. Interestingly, the reduction in suicide with lithium cannot be fully explained by lithium's ability to prevent episodes of depression. Although depression certainly contributes to the likelihood of suicide, impulsivity, agitation, and aggression also play a role. Experts speculate that lithium may modify one or more of the psychological or brain processes that give rise to suicide. Thus, lithium may have a place in the treatment of patients who are at high risk for suicide, whether or not they have manic-depressive illness.

I cannot leave the lithium/suicide story without mentioning lithium in drinking water. About a dozen studies, most conducted in the past decade, have shown with reasonable consistency that a relatively high concentration of lithium in a region's drinking water is associated with a relatively low rate of suicide.[31] These studies have been carried out in Texas, Japan, Austria, Greece, and elsewhere. There is no ready explanation for this association. The concentration of lithium in any drinking water is very low (a liter contains less than a thousandth of the smallest daily dose given as a treatment), so guzzling water, even when it contains relatively high amounts of lithium, results in serum lithium levels so tiny that it's hard to believe that they have any appreciable effect. One expert has suggested that even though the lithium imbibed with drinking water is insufficient to have any immediate psychological or biological effect, when taken over a long time it might.

The rationale for lithium use comes from hundreds of systematic studies, many of them controlled clinical trials, and the benefits of lithium are most often shown as an array of numbers and statistics: the percent of patients who get relief of symptoms, the proportion who stop having recurrences, the reduction in hospital stays, suicides, and health care costs. Impressive as these results are, they do not fully illustrate the impact of lithium on people's lives.

By the mid-1960s, Mogens Schou and Poul Baastrup were aware of lithium's potential to transform the lives of people with manic-depressive illness. When we look closely at the details of this transformation, at lithium's capacity to banish chaos, agony, and destruction from people's lives, it's not hard to understand Schou and Baastrup's reluctance to subject lithium to a placebo-controlled study, a study them to withhold lithium from people who could benefit so much from it. Shepherd and Blackwell were correct in some of their criticisms of Baastrup and Schou's "uncontrolled" initial prophylaxis study (see chapter 6) and in their insistence that definite proof of lithium's preventive value required a placebo-controlled investigation. But the humanitarian concerns that were behind Baastrup and Schou's reluctance to conduct such a study were not, as Shepherd implied, a trivial matter.

IN 1967, Robert Lowell started taking lithium. For 18 years, the celebrated poet had suffered with a brutal form of manic-depressive illness. None of the treatments he had undergone, and he had tried many, had reined in his yearly episodes of severe, destructive mania or his excruciating depressions. More often than not, these flare-ups culminated in a hospital stay. In 1968, about a year and a half after he started lithium, the novelist Richard Stern paid a visit to Lowell and recorded his observations:

"He showed me the bottle of lithium capsules. Another medical gift from Copenhagen. Had I heard what his trouble was? 'Salt deficiency.' This had been the first year in eighteen he hadn't had an attack. There'd been fourteen or fifteen of them over the past eighteen years. Frightful humiliation and waste. . . . His face seemed smoother, the weight of distress-attacks and anticipation both gone."[32]

Lowell went on to take lithium for the next eight years, and over that time was hospitalized for mania only once. Reflecting on lithium's impact, Lowell said: "It's terrible . . . to think that all I've suffered and all the suffering I've caused, might have arisen from the lack of a little salt in my brain."[33]

Decades later, in 2015, a freelance writer from Brooklyn named Jaime Lowe wrote a *New York Times Magazine* article titled "I Don't Believe in God, but I Believe in Lithium." In it Lowe described her 20-year struggle with manic-depressive illness and in particular her devastating manic episodes. She credited lithium with curbing those episodes (and her depressions), allowing her to live a "normal" life; she had a regular job and a long-term partner. At the time Lowe was facing the likelihood that because of kidney problems related to her lithium treatment, she would need to stop the lithium. The idea of being off lithium terrified her. She was terribly worried that her manic episodes would return, as they had 13 years previously, when she had briefly stopped taking lithium. "I worry that without lithium I will lose my job, my partner, my home, my mind."[34]

Lowe's story of a life rescued by lithium is not at all unusual. For 50 years, it has been the typical result of lithium treatment. Lithium made it possible for Mr. G, from this book's introduction, to live an ordinary life, working and indeed thriving in a mid-sized city rather than wandering the streets between stays in one psychiatric hospital or another.

As Lowe described in *Mental: Lithium, Love, and Losing My Mind*, the memoir that grew out of her article, after stopping lithium she did not have an easy time of it. Adhering to the standard approach for people who need to discontinue lithium, her doctor prescribed Depakote (a brand name for valproate). It gave her intolerable side effects; in addition to developing dry skin and nasty indigestion, she was irritable, depressed, and crying all the time. Sticking to the recommended guidelines, her doctor next suggested Tegretol, (a brand name for carbamazepine). Like valproate, carbamazepine is an antiseizure drug that has been shown to be of benefit in treating manic-depressive illness. No luck. After several weeks, blood tests showed that Tegretol was damaging her liver. At this point, Lowe seriously considered staying on lithium for the rest of her life, risking kidney failure and the necessity for dialysis. Experts she consulted suggested that she give Depakote another try. She did, and as luck would have it, the pharmacy that filled her prescription this time provided the Depakote in a slightly different formulation. She still suffered some unpleasant side effects, in particular indigestion and hair loss, but they were milder than before and bearable. After several months on Depakote and without lithium, Lowe was feeling okay both psychologically and physically. When we spoke recently, Lowe had been on Depakote for a year and a half. She has not yet suffered a manic or depressive episode, but it is too early to tell if Depakote will prevent future attacks as well as lithium did.[35]

THE LITHIUM story is not over. Starting with Cade's speculation in his original report that lithium treatment helps patients with mania because they have a deficiency in lithium, there has been no lack of theories accounting for lithium's benefits. Research continues on how it works. In the years since its discovery, scientists have accumulated a vast amount of information about lithium's effects on the brain. We know a lot about how it affects genes, cell membranes, and so-called cell signaling (a basic process mediated by enzymes, hormones, and other molecules that regulates the activity of neurons and other cells). Because lithium has such a unique and specific effect on manic-depressive illness, the hope persists that further understanding of what lithium does in the brain to alleviate manic symptoms and to prevent manic and depressive attacks will provide a crucial clue about the cause of manic-depressive illness. But as yet lithium's mechanism of action remains elusive.

We simply don't know which of lithium's innumerable biological effects accounts for its ability to prevent episodes of mania and depression. Part of the conundrum lies in the very multiplicity of cell processes altered by lithium. The other drugs used in psychiatry—much larger and more complex synthetic molecules—have fewer biological effects; and although we don't have a clear understanding of how these drugs alleviate symptoms, we do have enough clues to narrow the search to a few plausible mechanisms—something we don't have with lithium.

Contributing to our intractable ignorance of how lithium works is the inescapable fact that, notwithstanding Cade's and others' speculations, we simply don't have a clue about what causes manic-depressive illness, other than presuming that it has something to do with genes. Knowledge of how a drug works requires a clear understanding of the disease process that the drug targets. We know, for example, a good deal about the bodily processes that produce high blood pressure, including some of the enzymes and other chemicals involved, and that knowledge allows us to understand how the drugs that treat high blood pressure work. Likewise, we know that the cough and fever of pneumonia can result from a bacterial infection, and we know that antibiotics work by killing those bacteria. We don't yet have that sort of basic information about manic-depressive illness.

Over the years since Cade's discovery, lithium has been tried in essentially every psychiatric ailment, from schizophrenia to alcoholism. Disorders characterized (like manic-depressive illness) by episodic outbreaks, such as premenstrual syndrome (PMS), certain addictions, and recurrent aggressive outbursts, have been particularly tempting targets for lithium. But lithium has not proved effective in these conditions or in the other psychiatric conditions (apart from manic-depressive illness) in which hopeful investigators have tested it.

Given lithium's similarity to critical body chemicals—sodium, potassium, magnesium, and others—and its ability to displace these chemicals and affect cells throughout the body, it is no surprise that it has a variety of biological effects, some of which have potential value in the treatment of medical disease. For example, lithium shows antiviral activity in laboratory tests and seems to have some use in treating and preventing herpesvirus infections. Because lithium stimulates the production of infection-fighting white blood cells, it has been suggested as a remedy for the drop in such cells during cancer chemotherapy. Notwithstanding these and other treatment possibilities, as of now the only established medical role for lithium (aside from its role in the treatment of manic-depressive illness) is as one of the agents that prevent cluster headaches (unbearably severe, recurrent headaches).[36]

Still, lithium's therapeutic possibilities are far from exhausted. Research over the past two decades shows that lithium is "neuroprotective." It prevents damage to—and the death of—neurons and promotes nerve cell growth. Some experts believe that lithium's ability to preserve and foster the growth of nerve cells lies behind its capacity to alter the course of manic-depressive illness and to prevent episodes of mania and depression. But more closely tied to lithium's neuroprotective properties is a therapeutic possibility that opens up an entirely new treatment horizon; preliminary studies suggest that lithium may prevent dementia. Patients with bipolar illness who take lithium are less likely to develop dementia than those who don't, and a high lithium concentration in drinking water is also associated with a low prevalence of dementia.[37] Does lithium in fact ward off dementia? It's too early to tell. But the facts so far are sufficiently compelling to warrant further investigation.

It's not hard to imagine what John Cade would make of the recent observations on lithium and dementia. Given his experience in epidemiological research (remember the fruit trees?) and his awareness of important and intractable psychiatric problems, I see him at the head of the pack, launching a large-scale study of lithium and dementia throughout Victoria. Cade would be undeterred by the fact that as yet lithium has no place in the conventional understanding of dementia. You need to "test it and see," he would say.

This, of course, is only a guess. There is no way I could know what Cade would actually do. But if an obscure psychiatrist, working in isolation with little equipment and no research funds managed to come up with one of the most important treatment discoveries in psychiatry—in fact, in all of medicine—then who knows what else is possible?

Cade's intense curiosity, which seemed to extend to everything that came his way, certainly played a part in his contribution. He had a gift for accurate observation, for perception unaltered by preconceived notions of what he might find. Moreover, Cade seemed to have a propensity for divergent thinking—for free-flowing spontaneous association and making unexpected "nonlinear" connections. This cognitive style was certainly at play in his lithium research. So was persistence; he didn't give up at Changi or in his makeshift lab. Even his tendency to be highly disciplined and somewhat compulsive—seven daily cigarettes at regular intervals; morning tea, lunch, and afternoon tea at precisely the same times each day; and a glass of sherry every evening—may have contributed to his research success. And let's not forget genetics: Cade came from a long line of physicians and pharmacists; his paternal great-grandfather migrated from England and established one of the first pharmacies in Melbourne. I don't discount the possibility that a scientific bent was in his DNA.

But in the end I can't improve on what two of his colleagues wrote about him on the 50th anniversary of his lithium paper: "Changes in scientific method and the expansion of knowledge all make his kind of discovery far less possible . . . We may not know how to create such minds, but, when they become evident, we should accord them sanctuary for their enquiry. Such spirits cannot be decanted into a neat cost structure. The John Cades among us see, make inspired connections and extend a calming and healing hand."[38] We in the scientific community should keep an eye out for the Cades, and for the lithiums as well. Breakthroughs can still come from the unlikeliest of people and places.

ACKNOWLEDGMENTS

MY THANKS to those who, in email exchanges and interviews, generously provided me with information about the lithium story and allowed, indeed encouraged, me to pick their formidable brains. Many of them also sent me source documents not otherwise available: Jean Anderson, Ross Baldessarini, Tom Ban, Barry Blackwell, Jack Cade, Barney Carroll, Edmond Chiu, Neil Cole, Greg de Moore, Dave Dunner, Ron Fieve, David Healy, Neil Johnson, Norman Lear, Jacki Lindsay, Jaime Lowe, Gordon Parker, Johan Schioldann, Jason Sello, John A. Talbott, and Leonardo Tondo.

I am particularly indebted to Sam Gershon, himself a lithium pioneer, who talked with me about lithium for hours.

I am grateful to those who, without knowing me from Adam, went out of their way to find, copy, scan and do the other stuff necessary to provide me with critical documents: Jon Cullum, Michael Head, Jacky Healy, Russell Johnson, and Judy Sinclair.

I asked Richard Stamelman, a great friend for six decades, to translate French articles about lithium into English, and he willingly did so.

Ellen Welty helped get this book in final shape, compiling the notes, fact checking, and editing. It's a better book because of her.

My editors at Liveright Publishing, Katie Adams and Marie Pantojan, are more than good wordsmiths. They were supportive, considerate, and encouraging at every turn.

Jessica Papin, my agent, has been simply splendid. She shepherded this book—and me—with tact, kindness, and wisdom. It wouldn't have happened without her.

Gordon Brown, Matthew Brown, and Susan Brown encouraged and supported me through what turned out to be a long haul. Christine Ryan was unflagging in her love and support. She read and commented on each chapter as I finished it, and she cheered me on. I sought her counsel at every turn, and she always came through.

NOTES

Introduction

1. Mark W. Kirschner, Elizabeth Marincola, and Elizabeth Olmsted Teisberg, "The Role of Biomedical Research in Health Care Reform," *Science* 266, no. 5182 (1994): 49–51.
2. F. N. Johnson, "John F. J. Cade, 1912 to 1980: A Reminiscence," *Pharmacopsychiatria* 14 (1981): 148.
3. Johnson, "A Reminisence," 148.

1: Manic-Depressive Illness, A Brief History

1. John F. J. Cade, *Mending the Mind: A Short History of Twentieth Century Psychiatry* (Melbourne: Sun Books, 1979), 68.
2. Ludwig von Pastor, *The History of the Popes*, vol. 1, *The Great Schism*, 4th ed. (1913 Reprint: Morrisville, NC: Ghislieri Books, in conjunction with Lulu Press, 2015), 122.
3. Cade, *Mending the Mind*, 67–68.
4. Ronald Fieve, *Moodswing: Dr. Fieve on Depression* (New York: William Morrow, 1975).
5. Neel Burton, "A Short History of Bipolar Disorder," *Hide and Seek* (blog), *Psychology Today*, June 21, 2012, accessed April 18, 2016, https://www

.psychologytoday.com/blog/hide-and-seek/201206/short-history-bipolar
-disorder.

6. Thomas Willis, *Two Discourses Concerning the Soul of Brutes*, trans. Samuel
Pordage (London: Thomas Dring, 1683), 201, quoted in Frederick K.
Goodwin and Kay R. Jamison, *Manic-Depressive Illness: Bipolar Disorders
and Recurrent Depression*, 2nd ed. (New York: Oxford University Press,
2007), 6.

7. William Styron, *Darkness Visible: A Memoir of Madness* (New York: Random
House, 1990), 37.

8. Goodwin and Jamison, *Manic-Depressive Illness*, 419–21.

9. Janice A. Egeland et al., "Bipolar Affective Disorders Linked to DNA
Markers on Chromosome 11," *Nature* 325 (February 1987): 783–87.

10. Egeland et al., "Bipolar Affective Disorders," 783–87.

11. John R. Kelsoe et al., "Re-evaluation of the Linkage Relationship between
Chromosome 11p Loci and the Gene for Bipolar Affective Disorder in the
Old Order Amish," *Nature* 342, no. 18 (1989): 238–43.

12. Edward Shorter, *A History of Psychiatry: From the Era of the Asylum to the Age
of Prozac* (New York: John Wiley & Sons, 1997), 196.

13. Carlo Flascha, "On Opium: Its History, Legacy and Cultural Benefits," *Prospect Journal of International Affairs at UCSD*, May 25, 2011, accessed June 6,
2018, https://prospectjournal.org/2011/05/25/on-opium-its-history-legacy
-and-cultural-benefits/.

14. Flascha, "On Opium."

15. Shorter, *History of Psychiatry*, 1–2.

16. Cade, *Mending the Mind*, p. 68; Oliver D. Howes, Asha Khambhaita, and
Paolo Fusar-Poli, "Images in Psychiatry: Julius Wagner-Jauregg, 1857–
1940," *American Journal of Psychiatry* 166, no. 4 (2009): 409. https://ajp
.psychiatryonline.org/doi/pdf/10.1176/appi.ajp.2008.08081271.

17. Thomas Quinn Beesley, "When the Brain Is Sick," review of *The Defective,
Delinquent and Insane*, by Henry A. Cotton, *New York Times*, June 18, 1922.

18. Andrew Scull, *Madhouse: A Tragic Tale of Megalomania and Modern Medicine*
(New Haven, CT: Yale University Press, 2005).

19. Cade, *Mending the Mind*, 57.

20. Dominik Gross and Gereon Schäfer, "Egas Moniz (1874–1955) and the
'Invention' of Modern Psychosurgery: A Historical and Ethical Reanalysis
under Special Consideration of Portuguese Original Sources," *Journal of
Neurosurgery* 30, no. 2 (2011): 2–3.

21. Kay Redfield Jamison, *Touched with Fire. Manic-Depressive Illness and the Artistic Temperament* (New York: Free Press, 1993), 181.

22. Jamison, *Touched with Fire*, 181.

23. Ruth Richards et al., "Creativity in Manic-Depressives, Cyclothymes,

Their Normal Relatives, and Control Subjects," *Journal of Abnormal Psychology* 97, no. 3 (1988): 281–88.

2: The Naturalist

1. John F. J. Cade, "Contemporary Challenges in Psychiatry," *Australia & New Zealand Journal of Psychiatry* 5, no. 1 (1971): 16.
2. Johnson, "A Reminiscence," 149.
3. Greg de Moore and Ann Westmore, *Finding Sanity: John Cade, Lithium and the Taming of Bipolar Disorder* (Crow's Nest, Sydney, AU: Allen & Unwin, 2016), 244–45.
4. Cade, "Contemporary Challenges," 16.
5. De Moore and Westmore, *Finding Sanity*, 229.
6. Jack F. Cade, "John Frederick Joseph Cade: Family Memories on the Occasion of the 50th Anniversary of His Discovery of the Use of Lithium in Mania," *Australian & New Zealand Journal of Psychiatry* 33, no. 5 (1999): 617.
7. De Moore and Westmore, *Finding Sanity*, 111.
8. Author interview with Jack F. Cade, December 2017.
9. Jack F. Cade, "Family Memories," 615.
10. Jack F. Cade, "Family Memories," 618.
11. DeMoore and Westmore, *Finding Sanity*, 18.
12. Jack L. Evans, "Obituary for John Frederick Joseph Cade," *Australian & New Zealand Journal of Psychiatry* 15 (1980): 276.
13. John F. J. Cade, "Lecture 1: Research in Psychiatry: Lecture 1 of the Beattie-Smith Lectures," *Medical Journal of Australia* 2, no. 7 (1951): 219.
14. Cade, "Contemporary Challenges," 15.
15. Cade, *Mending the Mind*, 18.
16. F. M. Burnet, J. F. J. Cade, and Dora Lush, "The Serological Response to Influenza Virus Infection during an Epidemic, with Particular Reference to Subclinical Infection," *Medical Journal of Australia* 1, no. 12 (1940): 397–401.
17. Allan S. Walker, *Australia in the War*, vol. 1, *Clinical Problems of War* (Canberra, AU: Australian War Memorial, 1952), 705. Quoted in Ann Westmore and Greg de Moore, "The 'Mad Major' and His Idiosyncratic War: Linking Military Medicine and Lithium Therapy for Mania," *Health & History: Journal of the Australian & New Zealand Society for the History of Medicine* 15, no. 1 (2013): 21. Special issue: World War II and Medical Research in Australia.
18. Winston S. Churchill, *The Second World War*, vol. 4, *The Hinge of Fate* (New York: Bantam Books, 1962), 800.

19. Neil Cole and Gordon Parker, "Cade's Identification of Lithium for Manic-Depressive Illness—The Prospector Who Found a Gold Nugget," *Journal of Nervous and Mental Disease* 200, no. 12 (2012): 1102.

20. Churchill, *Hinge of Fate*, 87.

21. Westmore and de Moore, "The 'Mad Major'," 22.

22. Edmond Chiu and Rose-Marie Hegarty, "John Cade: The Man," *Australian & New Zealand Journal of Psychiatry* 33, supplement 1 (1999): S25.

23. Frederick Neil Johnson, *The History of Lithium Therapy* (London: Macmillan, 1984), 34.

24. Ann Westmore, "The Many Faces Of John Cade," in Johan Schioldann, *History of the Introduction of Lithium into Medicine and Psychiatry: Birth of Modern Psychopharmacology 1949* (Adelaide, AU: Adelaide Academic Press, 2009), 311.

3: Lithium

1. The report cited in this section is "Calculus in the Bladder, Treated by Litholysis, or Solution of the Stone by Injections of the Carbonate of Lithia, Conjoined with Lithotrity (Under the care of Mr. Ure)," *The Lancet* 2, no. 1930 (1860): 185–86. Two excellent sources on the history of lithium are Johnson's *History of Lithium Therapy* and Schioldann's *History of the Introduction of Lithium into Medicine and Psychiatry*.

2. William Alexander Hammond, *A Treatise on Diseases of the Nervous System* (New York: D. Appleton, 1871), 381.

3. Schioldann, *History of the Introduction of Lithium*, 78.

4. Alan D. Strobusch and James W. Jefferson, "The Checkered History of Lithium in Medicine," *Pharmacy in History* 22, no. 2 (1980): 73.

5. Strobusch and Jefferson, "The Checkered History," 73.

4: Breakthrough

1. Cade, "Lecture 1," 219.

2. Westmore and de Moore, "The 'Mad Major'," 37.

3. John F. Cade, "The Anticonvulsant Properties of Creatinine," *Medical Journal of Australia* 2 (November 1947): 621.

4. John F. J. Cade, "Lithium—Past, Present and Future," in *Lithium in Medical Practice*, eds. F. N. Johnson and S. Johnson (Lancaster, UK: MTP Press, 1978), 10.

5. John F. J. Cade, "The Story of Lithium," in *Discoveries in Biological Psychia-*

try, eds. Frank J. Ayd and Barry Blackwell (Baltimore: Ayd Medical Communications, 1984), 220.

6. Johnson, *History of Lithium Therapy*, 35.

7. Cade, "Story of Lithium," 221.

8. Cade, "Anticonvulsant Properties," 622. Cade found that pentamethylenetetrazol, a drug that induces convulsions, produced fatal convulsions in all the guinea pigs that got it, but creatinine prevented convulsions in half the animals. He then tried creatinine in at least one (human) patient who had epilepsy and frequent, almost daily, convulsions. Creatinine reduced the convulsions' frequency.

9. Cade, "Story of Lithium," 222.

10. Author interview with Jason Sello, September 2016.

11. Cade, "Story of Lithium," 222–23.

12. Cade, "Story of Lithium," 223.

13. Cade, "Lithium—Past, Present," 9–10.

14. Mogens Schou, "Lithium Perspectives," *Neuropsychobiology* 10 (1983): 9.

15. Cade, "Story of Lithium," 223.

16. Hammond, *A Treatise*, 381.

17. Vibram K. Yeragani and Samuel Gershon, "Hammond and Lithium: Historical Update," *Biological Psychiatry* 21, no. 11 (1986): 1101.

18. John F.J. Cade, "Lithium in Psychiatry: Historical Origins and Present Position," *Australia and New Zealand Journal of Psychiatry* 1 (1967): 61.

19. Chiu and Hegarty, "John Cade," S26.

20. Cade, "Lithium—Past, Present," 12.

21. Cade, "Lithium—Past, Present," 12–13.

22. Cade, "Story of Lithium," 223.

23. John F. J. Cade, "Lithium Salts in the Treatment of Psychotic Excitement," *Medical Journal of Australia* 2, no.10 (1949): 349–52.

24. Copies of Cade's original case notes of patient WB, courtesy of Bernard J. Carroll, email attachment to author, November 5, 2008.

25. Copies of Cade's original case notes of Patient WB, courtesy of Bernard J. Carroll, email attachment to author, November 5, 2008.

26. Brian Davies, "The First Patient to Receive Lithium," *Australian & New Zealand Journal of Psychiatry* 17, no. 4 (1983): 368.

27. Cade, "Story of Lithium," 223, 224; Cade, "Lithium—Past, Present," 12, 13.

28. Schioldann, *History of the Introduction of Lithium*, 244.

29. Johnson, *History of Lithium Therapy*, 41.

30. Roslyn Ross, "New Key to Mental Health," *Australian Women's Weekly*, May 13, 1970, p. 15.

31. Schioldann, *History of the Introduction of Lithium*, 290.

32. Barry Blackwell, Reply to Gershon by Blackwell, INHN, "The Lithium Controversy: A Historical Autopsy," February 19, 2015, accessed July 7, 2015, http://inhn.org/controversies/barry-blackwell-the-lithium-controversy-a-historical-autopsy/comment-by-samuel-gershon/reply-to-gershon-by-blackwell.html.

33. Barry Blackwell's comment on the interaction between Samuel Gershon and Gordon Johnson, INHN, "The Lithium Controversy," May 7, 2015, accessed July 7, 2015, http://inhn.org/controversies/barry-blackwell-the-lithium-controversy-a-historical-autopsy/barry-blackwells-comment-on-the-interaction-between-samuel-gershon-and-gordon-johnsson.html.

34. Mogens Schou, "Lithium treatment at 52," *Journal of Affective Disorders* 67, nos. 1–3 (2001): 22.

35. "John Frederick Joseph Cade: Obituary," *Medical Journal of Australia* 1 (1981): 489.

36. Cade, "Lithium Salts," 351.

37. Cade, "Lithium Salts," 352.

38. Evans, "Obituary," 276.

39. Cade, "Lecture 1," 215.

40. Johnson, "A Reminiscence," 149.

41. Cade, "Lithium Salts," 350.

5: Aftermath

1. Cade, "Story of Lithium," 219.

2. Johnson, *History of Lithium Therapy*, 48.

3. "Salt Substitute Kills 4, AMA Says," *New York Times*, February 19, 1949, Business sec.

4. John H. Talbott, "Use of Lithium Salts as a Substitute for Sodium Chloride," *Archives of Internal Medicine* 85, no. 1 (1950): 1–10.

5. Author interview with John A. Talbott (John Talbott's son), January 2017.

6. Talbott, "Use of Lithium Salts," 8.

7. Phil Gunby, "John H. Talbott, MD: 10th *JAMA* Editor," *Journal of the American Medical Association* 264, no. 17 (1990): 2183–84.

8. Talbott, "Use of Lithium Salts," 7.

9. Talbott, "Use of Lithium Salts," 8.

10. Johnson, *History of Lithium Therapy*, 161.

11. C. H. Noack and E. M. Trautner, "The Lithium Treatment of Maniacal Psychosis," *Medical Journal of Australia* 2, no. 7 (1951): 219.

12. Noack and Trautner, "The Lithium Treatment," 222.

13. Johnson, *History of Lithium Therapy*, 61.

14. Ulrich Schäfer, "Past and Present Conceptions Concerning the Use of Lithium in Medicine," *Journal of Trace and Microprobe Techniques* 16, no. 4 (1998): 539.

15. Mogens Schou, "Lithium: Personal Reminiscences," *Psychiatric Journal of the University of Ottawa* 14, no. 1 (1989): 261.

16. David Healy, *The Psychopharmacologists*, vol. 2 (London: Chapman & Hall, 1998), 264.

17. M. Schou et al., "The Treatment of Manic Psychoses by the Administration of Lithium Salts," *Journal of Neurology, Neurosurgery, and Psychiatry* 17, no. 4 (1954): 251.

18. Schou et al., "Treatment of Manic Psychoses," 256.

19. Schou et al., "Treatment of Manic Psychoses," 254.

20. Healy, *Psychopharmacologists*, 263.

21. Healy, *Psychopharmacologists*, 264.

22. Mogens Schou, "My Journey with Lithium," in Johan Schioldann, *History of the Introduction of Lithium into Medicine and Psychiatry: Birth of Modern Psychopharmacology 1949* (Adelaide, AU: Adelaide Academic Press, 2009), 314.

23. Mogens Schou, "Therapeutic and Toxic Properties of Lithium," in *Proceedings of the First International Congress of Neuropharmacology, Rome, September 1958*, eds. Philip Bradley, Pierre Deniker, and Corneille Raduoco-Thomas (Amsterdam: Elsevier, 1959): 687.

24. B. Glesinger, "Evaluation of Lithium in Treatment of Psychotic Excitement," *Medical Journal of Australia* 41 (February 1954): 278.

25. Glesinger, "Evaluation of Lithium," 280. Cade, as it happens, agreed at first that measuring serum lithium levels was an unnecessary frill; he felt that any competent clinician could manage the threat of toxicity simply by watching patients carefully, and he expressed this belief as late as 1969, sticking to it long after serum level monitoring had gained wide acceptance. Only in the very last papers he wrote about lithium, published in 1975 and 1978, did Cade finally acknowledge the value of regular serum lithium measurement. It is now the standard practice.

26. Max Margulies, "Suggestions for the Treatment of Schizophrenia and Manic-Depressive Patients," *Medical Journal of Australia* 35, no. 1 (1955): 137–41.

27. Cade, "The Story of Lithium," 219.

28. Johnson, *History of Lithium Therapy*, 58–9.

29. Johnson, *History of Lithium Therapy*, 105.

30. David Rice, "The Use of Lithium Salts in the Treatment of Manic States," *Journal of Mental Science* 102 (July 1956): 604–11.

31. Johnson, *History of Lithium Therapy*, 105.

32. Ronald Maggs, "Treatment of Manic Illness with Lithium Carbonate," *British Journal of Psychiatry* 109 (1963): 56–65.

33. Mogens Schou, "Lithium in Psychiatric Therapy: Stock-Taking after Ten Years," *Psychopharmacologia* 1 (1959): 76.

34. Mogens Schou, "General Discussion," in *Neuro-psychopharmacology,* vol. 3, *Proceedings of the Third Meeting of the Collegium Internationale Neuropsychopharmacologicum,* eds. P. B. Bradley, F. Flügel, and P. H. Hoch (Amsterdam: Elsevier, 1964), 591.

35. Schou, "General Discussion," 591.

6: Prophylaxis Rex

1. G. P. Hartigan, "Experiences of Treatment with Lithium Salts," in F. Neil Johnson, *The History of Lithium Therapy* (London: Macmillan Press, 1984), 185.

2. Hartigan, "Experiences of Treatment," 186.

3. Johnson, *History of Lithium Therapy,* 72.

4. Johnson, *History of Lithium Therapy,* 72.

5. Johnson, *History of Lithium Therapy,* 73.

6. Johnson, *History of Lithium Therapy,* 73.

7. Hartigan, "Experiences of Treatment," 183–87.

8. Johnson, *History of Lithium Therapy,* 75.

9. Johnson, *History of Lithium Therapy,* 71.

10. Poul Chr. Baastrup, "The Use of Lithium in Manic-Depressive Psychosis," *Comprehensive Psychiatry* 5, no. 6 (1964): 396–408.

11. Mogens Schou, "Normothymotics, 'Mood-Normalizers: Are Lithium and the Imipramine Drugs Specific for Affective Disorders?'" *British Journal of Psychiatry* 109 (1963): 803–09.

12. Johnson, *History of Lithium Therapy,* 77.

13. Poul Christian Baastrup and Mogens Schou, "Lithium as a Prophylactic Agent: Its Effect Against Recurrent Depressions and Manic-Depressive Psychosis," *Archives of General Psychiatry* 16 (February 1967): 171.

14. Burt Angrist, "Sam Gershon's Research Unit in Bellevue Hospital in New York," in *The History of Psychopharmacology and the CINP, As Told in Autobiography,* vol. 2, *The Triumph of Psychopharmacology and the Story of CINP,* eds. Thomas A. Ban, David Healy, and Edward Shorter (Budapest: Animula, 2000), 250–51 and 254.

15. Ronald R. Fieve, "Lithium: From Introduction to Public Awareness," in *The History of Psychopharmacology and the CINP, As Told in Autobiography,* vol. 2, *The Triumph Of Psychopharmacology and the Story of CINP,* eds. Thomas A. Ban, David Healy, and Edward Shorter (Budapest: Animula, 2000), 258.

16. Fieve, "Lithium: From Introduction," 259.

17. Author interview with John A. Talbott, January 2017.

18. Fieve, "Lithium: From Introduction," 259.

19. P. H. Blachly, "FDA vs. Physician: Does the Physician Have a Moral Obligation to Civil Disobedience?" *Psychiatric Opinion* 7 (August 1970): 34.

20. Les Brown, "Lithium Use in 'Maude.'" *New York Times*, January 22, 1976, Arts sec., 152.

21. Author interview with David Dunner, December 2015.

22. Patty Duke and Gloria Hochman, *A Brilliant Madness: Living With Manic-Depressive Illness* (New York: Bantam Books, 1993), 142.

23. Author interview with Ronald Fieve, May 2017.

24. Hannah Jane Parkinson, "Does Homeland Sensationalise Carrie Mathison's Bipolar Disorder?" *The Guardian*, December 1, 2014, accessed July 16, 2018, https://www.theguardian.com/commentisfree/2014/dec/01/homeland -carrie-mathison-bipolar-disorder-claire-danes.

25. Healy, *Psychopharmacologists*, 249.

26. Healy, *Psychopharmacologists*, 249.

27. Healy, *Psychopharmacologists*, 268.

28. Schou, "My Journey," 316.

29. Poul Christian Baastrup and Mogens Schou, "Prophylactic Lithium," *Lancet* 291, no. 7557 (1968): 1419–22.

30. William Sargant, letter to the editor, "Prophylactic Lithium?" *Lancet* 292, no. 7561 (1968), 216.

31. Brian Barraclough, "Felix Post," in *Talking About Psychiatry,* ed. Greg Wilkinson (London: Gaskell, Royal College of Psychiatrists, 1993), 167.

32. Healy, *Psychopharmacologists*, 272.

33. Schou, "My Journey," 316; Mogens Schou, "The Rise of Lithium Treatment in the 1960s," in *The History of Psychopharmacology and the CINP, As Told in Autobiography*, vol. 1, *The Rise of Psychopharmacology and the Story of CINP*, 2nd ed., eds. Thomas A. Ban, David Healy, and Edward Shorter (Vienna: Collegium Internationale Neuro-Psychopharmacologicum, 2010), 97.

34. Schou, "My Journey," 316; Schou, "The Rise of Lithium Treatment," 97.

35. Schou, "My Journey," 317.

36. Schou, "My Journey," 317.

37. P. C. Baastrup et al., "Prophylactic Lithium: Double-Blind Discontinuation in Manic-Depressive and Recurrent-Depressive Disorders," *Lancet* 2, no. 7668 (1970): 326–30.

38. Johnson, *History of Lithium Therapy,* 91.

39. Paul Grof, "Mogens Schou (1918–2005)," *Neuropsychopharmacology* 31, no. 4 (2006): 891.

40. Johnson, *History of Lithium Therapy*, 89.

41. Johnson, *History of Lithium Therapy*, 89.

42. Jules Angst, email message to author, September 28, 2017; comment by Paul Grof and Jules Angst: Reply to Barry Blackwell, INHN, "The Lithium Controversy: Somewhat Different Hindsights," January 2, 2015. http://inhn.org/cn/controversies/622/comment-by-paul-grof-and-jules -angst.html.

43. Mogens Schou, "Ethical Problems of Therapeutic and Prophylactic Trials in Manic-Depressive Disorder," in *Psihofarmakologija* 3, eds. N. Bohacek and M. Mihovilovic (Zagreb, Croatia: Med Naklada, 1974), 329.

44. Johan Schioldann, "John Cade's Seminal Lithium Paper Turns Fifty," editorial in *Acta Psychiatrica Scandinavica* (December 1999): 403.

Epilogue

1. De Moore and Westmore, *Finding Sanity,* 218.

2. Johnson, "A Reminiscence," 149.

3. Cade, "Story of Lithium," 225.

4. Cade, "Story of Lithium," 226.

5. Cade, "Story of Lithium," 228–29.

6. Cade, "Story of Lithium," 218–29.

7. Schioldann, *History of the Introduction of Lithium,* 263.

8. J. F. J. Cade, "The Metabolism of Melancholia," *Australian & New Zealand Journal of Psychiatry* 1, no. 23 (1967): 28.

9. Schou, "Lithium Perspectives," 8–9.

10. John F. J. Cade, "The Aetiology of Schizophrenia," *Medical Journal of Australia* 2 (July 1956): 138.

11. John F. J. Cade, "Manganese and Mongolism," *Medical Journal of Australia* 2 (1958): 848–49.

12. "Bernard Carroll," interview with Leo E. Hollister and Thomas A. Ban, in *An Oral History of Neuropsychopharmacology. The First Fifty Years. Peer Interviews,* ed. T. A. Ban, vol. 5, *Neuropsychopharmacology,* Samuel Gershon, ed. (Los Angeles: American College of Neuropsychopharmacology, 2011), 99.

13. Earl Arnett, "Discoveries In Biological Psychiatry Is Subject of Symposium," *Baltimore Sun,* April 17, 1970, 15.

14. Cade, "Lecture 1," 215.

15. Cade, "Lecture 1," 215.

16. Cade, "Lecture 1," 215.

17. John F. J. Cade, writing as Mensana, "Why Not Sleep Soundly?" *Messenger,* January 1, 1952.

18. John F. J. Cade, writing as Mensana, "Bringing Up Children," *Messenger,* December 1, 1951.

19. Cade, *Mending the Mind*, 90.

20. John F. J. Cade, writing as Mensana, "The Demon of Doubt," *Messenger*, March 1, 1952.

21. John F. J. Cade, "Masturbational Madness: An Historical Annotation," *Australian & New Zealand Journal of Psychiatry* 7, no. 23 (1973): 23.

22. John F. J. Cade, "An Eclectic Psychiatrist Looks at Homosexuality," in *Geigy Psychiatric Symposium*, ed. Neil McConaghy, vol. 2, *Liberation Movements and Psychiatry* (Sydney: Ciba-Geigy, 1974), 99.

23. Cade, "An Eclectic Psychiatrist," 99.

24. Schioldann, *History of the Introduction of Lithium*, 261.

25. Schou, "Lithium Perspectives," 9.

26. Frederick Neil Johnson, email message to author, October 18, 2015.

27. Cade, *Mending the Mind*, 75.

28. Kirschner et al., "The Role of Biomedical Research," 49.

29. Allan H. Young and Judith M. Hammond, "Lithium in Mood Disorders: Increasing Evidence Base, Declining Use?" *British Journal Of Psychiatry* 191 (December 2007): 474.

30. Young and Hammond, "Lithium in Mood Disorders," 474; Leonardo Tondo and Ross J. Baldessarini, "Antisuicidal Effects in Mood Disorders: Are They Unique to Lithium?" *Pharmacopsychiatry* 51 (April 2018): 177–88. doi: 10.1055/a-0596-7853; Andrea Cipriani et al., "Lithium in the Prevention of Suicide in Mood Disorders: Updated Systematic Review and Meta-Analysis," *British Medical Journal* 346, no. f3646 (2013). doi.org/10.1136/bmj.f3646.

31. Tondo and Baldessarini, "Antisuicidal Effects."

32. Goodwin and Jamison, *Manic-Depressive Illness*, 721; Ian Hamilton, *Robert Lowell: A Biography* (New York: Random House, 1982), 370.

33. Goodwin and Jamison, *Manic-Depressive Illness*, 699; Robert Giroux, ed., *Robert Lowell Collected Prose* (New York: Farrar, Straus, Giroux, 1967), xiii–xiv.

34. Jaime Lowe, "I Don't Believe in God, but I Believe in Lithium: My 20-Year Struggle with Bipolar Disorder," *New York Times Magazine*, Mental Health Issue (June 28, 2015), 62.

35. Author interview with Jaime Lowe, July 2018.

36. Tom Bschor, Ute Lewitzka, and Mazda Adli, "The Use of Lithium in Non-Psychiatric Conditions," in *Lithium in Neuropsychiatry: The Comprehensive Guide*, eds. Michael Bauer, Paul Grof, and Bruno Müller-Oerlinghausen (Abingdon, UK: Informa UK, 2006), 237–39.

37. James Gallagher, "Lithium in Tap Water May Cut Dementia," BBC News, Health sec., August 24, 2017. http://www.bbc.com/news/health -41024697; Anna Fels, "Should We All Take a Bit of Lithium?" *New York*

Times, Sunday Review, Sept 14, 2014, SR6; Lars Vedel Kessing et al, "Association of Lithium in Drinking Water with the Incidence of Dementia," *JAMA Psychiatry*, 74, no. 10 (2017): 1005–10.

38. Philip B. Mitchell and Dusan Hadzi-Pavlovic, "John Cade and the Discovery of Lithium Treatment for Manic Depressive Illness," *Medical Journal of Australia*, 171, no. 6 (1999): 264.

SELECTED BIBLIOGRAPHY

Angrist, Burt. "Sam Gershon's Research Unit in Bellevue Hospital in New York." In *The History of Psychopharmacology and the CINP, As Told in Autobiography*, Vol. 2, *The Triumph of Psychopharmacology and the Story of CINP*, edited by Thomas A. Ban, David Healy, and Edward Shorter, 250–54. Budapest: Animula, 2000.

Arnett, Earl. "Discoveries In Biological Psychiatry Subject of Symposium." *Baltimore Sun*, April 17, 1970.

Baastrup, Poul Christian. "The Use of Lithium in Manic-Depressive Psychosis." *Comprehensive Psychiatry* 5, no. 6 (1964): 396–408.

Baastrup, Poul Christian, and Mogens Schou. "Lithium as a Prophylactic Agent: Its Effect Against Recurrent Depressions and Manic-Depressive Psychosis." *Archives of General Psychiatry* 16 (February 1967): 162–72.

Baastrup, Poul Christian, and Mogens Schou. "Prophylactic Lithium." *The Lancet* 291, no. 7557 (1968): 1419–22.

Baastrup, Poul Christian, J. C. Poulsen, M. Schou, K. Thomsen, and A. Amdisen. "Prophylactic Lithium: Double-Blind Discontinuation in Manic-Depressive and Recurrent-Depressive Disorders." *The Lancet* 2, no. 7668 (1970): 326–30.

Ban, Thomas A., David Healy, and Edward Shorter, eds. *The History of Psychopharmacology and the CINP, As Told in Autobiography*, Vol. 2, *The Triumph of Psychopharmacology and the Story of CINP*. Budapest: Animula, 2000.

Barraclough, Brian. "Felix Post." In *Talking About Psychiatry*, edited by Greg

Wilkinson, 157–77. London: Gaskell, Royal College of Psychiatrists, 1993.

Beesley, Thomas Quinn. "When the Brain is Sick." Review of *The Defective, Delinquent and Insane*, by Henry A. Cotton, *New York Times*, June 18, 1922.

"Bernard Carroll." Leo E. Hollister and Thomas A. Ban, interviewers. In *An Oral History of Neuropsychopharmacology. The First Fifty Years. Peer Interviews*, edited by Thomas A. Ban. Vol. 5, *Neuropsychopharmacology*, edited by Samuel Gershon, 85–102. Los Angeles: American College of Neuropsychopharmacology, 2011.

Blachly, P. H. "FDA vs. Physician: Does the Physician Have a Moral Obligation to Civil Disobedience?" *Psychiatric Opinion* 7 (August 1970): 29–35.

Brown, Les. "Lithium Use in 'Maude.'" *New York Times*, January 22, 1976, Arts sec.

Bschor, Tom, Ute Lewitzka, and Mazda Adli. "The Use of Lithium in Non-Psychiatric Conditions." In *Lithium in Neuropsychiatry: The Comprehensive Guide*, edited by Michael Bauer, Paul Grof, and Bruno Müller-Oerlinghausen, 237–50. Abingdon, UK: Informa UK, 2006.

Burnet, Frank M., John F. J. Cade, and Dora Lush. "The Serological Response to Influenza Virus Infection During an Epidemic, with Particular Reference to Subclinical Infection." *Medical Journal of Australia* 1, no. 12 (1940): 397–401.

Burton, Neel. "A Short History of Bipolar Disorder." *Hide and Seek* (blog). June 21, 2012. Accessed April 18, 2016, https://www.psychologytoday.com/blog/hide-and-seek/201206/short-history-bipolar-disorder.

Cade, Jack F. "John Frederick Joseph Cade: Family Memories on the Occasion of the 50th Anniversary of His Discovery of the Use of Lithium in Mania." *Australian & New Zealand Journal of Psychiatry* 33, no. 5 (1999): 615–18.

Cade, John F. "The Aetiology of Schizophrenia." *Medical Journal of Australia* 2 (1956): 135–39.

Cade, John F. J. "The Anticonvulsant Properties of Creatinine." *Medical Journal of Australia*, 2 (1947): 621–23.

Cade, John F. J. "Contemporary Challenges in Psychiatry." *Australian & New Zealand Journal of Psychiatry* 5, no. 1 (1971): 10–17.

Cade, John F. J. "An Eclectic Psychiatrist Looks at Homosexuality." In *Geigy Psychiatric Symposium*, Vol. 2, *Liberation Movements and Psychiatry*, edited by Neil McConaghy, 99–101. St. Leonards, AU: Ciba-Geigy, 1974.

Cade, John F. J. "Lithium—Past, Present and Future." In *Lithium in Medical Practice*, edited by F. N. Johnson and S. Johnson, 5–16. Lancaster, UK: MTP Press, 1978.

Cade, John F. J. "Lithium in Psychiatry: Historical Origins and Present Position." *Australian & New Zealand Journal of Psychiatry* 1 (1967): 61–62.

Cade, John F. J. "Lithium Salts in the Treatment of Psychotic Excitement." *Medical Journal of Australia* 2, no. 10 (1949): 349–52.

Cade, John F. J. "Manganese and Mongolism." *Medical Journal of Australia* 2 (December 1958): 848–49.

Cade, John F. J. "Masturbational Madness: An Historical Annotation." *Australian & New Zealand Journal of Psychiatry* 7 (1973): 23–26.

Cade, John F. J. *Mending the Mind: A Short History of Twentieth Century Psychiatry.* Melbourne: Sun Books, 1979.

Cade, John F. J. "The Metabolism of Melancholia." *Australian & New Zealand Journal of Psychiatry* 1, no. 23 (1967): 23–29.

Cade, John F. J., writing as Mensana. "A Psychiatrist Asks . . . Why Not Sleep Soundly." *The Messenger*, January 1, 1952, 43–44.

Cade, John F. J., writing as Mensana. "A Psychiatrist Writes for the Scrupulous . . . The Demon of Doubt." *The Messenger*, March 1, 1952, 177–79.

Cade, John F. J., writing as Mensana. "A Psychiatrist Writes on . . . Bringing Up Children." *The Messenger*, December 1, 1951, 788–89.

Cade, John F. J. "Research in Psychiatry: Lecture 1 of The Beattie-Smith Lectures." *Medical Journal of Australia* 2, no. 7 (1951): 213–19.

Cade, John F. J. "The Story of Lithium." In *Discoveries in Biological Psychiatry*, edited by Frank J. Ayd and Barry Blackwell, 218–29. 2nd ed. Baltimore: Ayd Medical Communications, 1984.

"Calculus in the Bladder, Treated by Litholysis, or Solution of the Stone by Injections of the Carbonate of Lithia, Conjoined with Lithotrity (Under the care of Mr. Ure)." *The Lancet* 2, no. 1930 (1860): 185–86.

Chiu, Edmond, and Rose-Marie Hegarty. "John Cade: The Man." *Australian & New Zealand Journal of Psychiatry* 33, supplement (1999): S24–26.

Churchill, Winston S. *The Second World War*, Vol. 4, *The Hinge of Fate*. New York: Bantam Books, 1962.

Cipriani, Andrea, Keith Hawton, Sarah Stockton, and John R. Geddes. "Lithium in the Prevention of Suicide in Mood Disorders: Updated Systematic Review and Meta-analysis." *British Medical Journal* 346, no. f3646 (2013): 1–13. https://www.bmj.com/content/346/bmj.f3646.

Cole, Neil, and Gordon Parker. "Cade's Identification of Lithium for Manic-Depressive Illness—The Prospector Who Found a Gold Nugget." *The Journal of Nervous and Mental Disease* 200, no. 12 (2012): 1101–104.

Davies, Brian. "The First Patient to Receive Lithium." *Australian & New Zealand Journal of Psychiatry* 17, no. 4 (1983): 366–68.

De Moore, Greg, and Ann Westmore. *Finding Sanity: John Cade, Lithium and the Taming of Bipolar Disorder.* Crow's Nest, Sydney, AU: Allen & Unwin, 2016.

Duke, Patty, and Gloria Hochman. *A Brilliant Madness: Living with Manic-Depressive Illness.* New York: Bantam Books, 1993.

Egeland, Janice A., Daniela S. Gerhard, David L. Pauls, James N. Sussex, Kenneth K. Kidd, Cleona R. Allen, Abram M. Hostetter, and David E. Housman. "Bipolar Affective Disorders Linked to DNA Markers on Chromosome 11." *Nature* 325 (February 1987): 783–87.

Evans, Jack L., "Obituary for John Frederick Joseph Cade." *Australian & New Zealand Journal of Psychiatry* 15 (1980): 275–77.

Fels, Anna. "Should We All Take a Bit of Lithium?" *New York Times*, Sunday Review, opinion section, Sept 14, 2014, SR6.

Fieve, Ronald R. "Lithium: From Introduction to Public Awareness." In *The History of Psychopharmacology and the CINP, As Told in Autobiography*, Vol. 2, *The Triumph of Psychopharmacology and the Story of CINP*, edited by Thomas A. Ban, David Healy, and Edward Shorter, 258–60. Budapest: Animula, 2000.

Fieve, Ronald R. *Moodswing: Dr. Fieve on Depression.* New York: William Morrow, 1975.

Flascha, Carlo. "On Opium: Its History, Legacy and Cultural Benefits." *Prospect Journal of International Affairs at UCSD*, May 25, 2011, accessed June 6, 2018, https://prospectjournal.org/2011/05/25/on-opium-its-history-legacy-and-cultural-benefits/

Gallagher, James. "Lithium in Tap Water May Cut Dementia." BBC News, health sec., August 24, 2017. http://www.bbc.com/news/health-41024697.

Glesinger, Bernard. "Evaluation of Lithium in Treatment of Psychotic Excitement." *Medical Journal of Australia* 41 (February 1954): 277–83.

Goodwin, Frederick K., and Kay Redfield Jamison. *Manic-Depressive Illness: Bipolar Disorders and Recurrent Depression.* 2nd ed. New York: Oxford University Press, 2007.

Grof, Paul. "Mogens Schou (1918–2005): Obituary." *Neuropsychopharmacology* 31, no. 4 (2006): 891–92.

Gross, Dominik, and Gereon Schäfer. "Egas Moniz (1874–1955) and the 'Invention' of Modern Psychosurgery: A Historical and Ethical Reanalysis under Special Consideration of Portuguese Original Sources." *Journal of Neurosurgery* 30, no. 2 (2011): 1–7.

Gunby, Phil. "John H. Talbott, MD: 10th *JAMA* Editor." In *Journal of the American Medical Association*, obituaries, 264, no. 17 (1990): 2183–84.

Hamilton, Ian. *Robert Lowell: A Biography.* New York: Random House, 1982.

Hammond, William Alexander. *A Treatise on Diseases of the Nervous System.* New York: D. Appleton and Company, 1871.

Hartigan, G. P. "Experiences of Treatment with Lithium Salts." In *The History of Lithium Therapy*, edited by F. Neil Johnson, 183–87. London: Macmillan Press, 1984.

Hartigan, G. P. "The Use of Lithium Salts in Affective Disorders." *British Journal of Psychiatry* 109 (1963): 810–14.

Healy, David. *The Psychopharmacologists.* Vol. 2. London: Chapman & Hall, 1998.

Jamison, Kay Redfield. *Touched with Fire. Manic-Depressive Illness and the Artistic Temperament.* New York: Free Press, 1993.

"John Frederick Joseph Cade: Obituary." *Medical Journal of Australia.* 1 (1981): 489.

Johnson, Frederick Neil. *The History of Lithium Therapy.* London: Macmillan, 1984.

Johnson, Frederick Neil. "John F. J. Cade, 1912 to 1980: A Reminiscence." *Pharmacopsychiatria* 14 (1981): 148–49.

Johnson, Frederick Neil, and Susan Johnson, eds. *Lithium in Medical Practice.* Lancaster, UK: MTP Press, 1978.

Kelsoe, John R., Edward I. Ginns, Janice A. Egeland, Daniela S. Gerhard, Alisa M. Goldstein, Sherri J. Bale, David L. Pauls, Robert T. Long, Kenneth Kidd, and Giovanni Conte. "Re-evaluation of the Linkage Relationship between Chromosome 11p Loci and the Gene for Bipolar Affective Disorder in the Old Order Amish." *Nature* 342, no. 18 (1989): 238–43.

Kessing, Lars Vedel, Thomas Alexander Gerds, Nikoline Nygard Knudsen, Lisbeth Flindt Jørgensen, Søren Munch Kristiansen, Denitza Voutchkova, Vibeke Ernsten, Jörg Schullehner, Birgitte Hansen, Per Kragh Andersen et al. "Association of Lithium in Drinking Water with the Incidence of Dementia." *JAMA Psychiatry* 74, no. 10 (2017): 1005–10.

Kirschner, Mark W., Elizabeth Marincola, and Elizabeth Olmsted Teisberg. "The Role of Biomedical Research in Health Care Reform." *Science* 266, no. 5182 (1994): 49–51.

Lowe, Jaime. "I Don't Believe in God, but I Believe in Lithium: My 20-Year Struggle with Bipolar Disorder." *New York Times Magazine*, June 28, 2015, Mental Health Issue, 62.

Lowell, Robert. *Robert Lowell Collected Prose*, edited by Robert Giroux. New York: Farrar, Straus, Giroux, 1987.

Maggs, Ronald. "Treatment of Manic Illness with Lithium Carbonate." *British Journal of Psychiatry* 109 (1963): 56–65.

Margulies, Max. "Suggestions for the Treatment of Schizophrenic and Manic-Depressive Patients." *Medical Journal of Australia* 35, no. 1 (1955): 137–41.

Mitchell, Philip B., and Dusan Hadzi-Pavlovic. "John Cade and the Discovery of Lithium Treatment for Manic Depressive Illness." *Medical Journal of Australia* 171, no. 5 (1999): 262–64.

Noack, C. H., and E. M. Trautner. "The Lithium Treatment of Maniacal Psychosis." *Medical Journal of Australia* 2, no. 7 (1951): 219–22.

Parkinson, Hannah Jane. "Does Homeland Sensationalise Carrie Mathison's Bipolar Disorder?" *The Guardian*, December 1, 2014, accessed July 16, 2018, https://www.theguardian.com/commentisfree/2014/dec/01/homeland-carrie-mathison-bipolar-disorder-claire-danes.

Pastor, Ludwig von. *The History of the Popes*, Vol. 1, *The Great Schism*. 4th ed. 1913 Reprint, Morrisville, NC: Ghislieri Books, in conjunction with Lulu Press, 2015.

Rice, David. "The Use of Lithium Salts in the Treatment of Manic States." *Journal of Mental Science* 102 (July 1956): 604–11.

Richards, Ruth, Dennis K. Kinney, Inge Lunde, Maria Benet, and Ann P. C. Merzel. "Creativity in Manic-Depressives, Cyclothymes, Their Normal Relatives, and Control Subjects." *Journal of Abnormal Psychology* 97, no. 3 (1988): 281–88.

Ross, Roslyn. "New Key to Mental Health." *Australian Women's Weekly*, May 13, 1970, 15.

"Salt Substitute Kills 4, AMA Says." *New York Times*, February 19, 1949, Business sec.

Sargant, William. Letter to the editor, "Prophylactic Lithium?" *The Lancet* 292, no. 7561 (1968), 216.

Schäfer, Ulrich. "Past and Present Conceptions Concerning the Use of Lithium in Medicine." *Journal of Trace and Microprobe Techniques* 16, no. 4 (1998): 535–56.

Schioldann, Johan. Invited guest editorial, "John Cade's Seminal Lithium Paper Turns Fifty." *Acta Psychiatrica Scandinavica*100 (1999): 403–404.

Schioldann, Johan. *History of the Introduction of Lithium into Medicine and Psychiatry: Birth of Modern Psychopharmacology 1949*. Adelaide, AU: Adelaide Academic Press, 2009.

Schou, Mogens. "Ethical Problems of Therapeutic and Prophylactic Trials in Manic-Depressive Disorder." In *Psihofarmakologija* 3, edited by N. Bohacek and M. Mihovilovic, 323–32. Zagreb, Croatia: Med Naklada, 1974.

Schou, Mogens. "General Discussion." In *Neuro-psychopharmacology*, Vol. 3, *Proceedings of the Third Meeting of the Collegium Internationale Neuropsychopharmacologicum*, edited by P. B. Bradley, F. Flügel, and P. H. Hoch, 591. Amsterdam: Elsevier, 1964.

Schou, Mogens. "Lithium: Personal Reminiscences." *Psychiatric Journal of the University of Ottawa* 14, no. 1 (1989): 260–62.

Schou, Mogens. "Lithium in Psychiatric Therapy: Stock-taking after ten years." *Psychopharmacologia* 1 (1959): 65–78.

Schou, Mogens. "Lithium Perspectives." *Neuropsychobiology* 10 (1983): 7–12.

Schou, Mogens. "Lithium Treatment at 52." *Journal of Affective Disorders* 67, nos. 1–3 (2001): 21–32.

Schou, Mogens. "My Journey with Lithium." In Johan Schioldann, *History of the Introduction of Lithium into Medicine and Psychiatry: Birth of Modern Psychopharmacology 1949*, 313–20. Adelaide, AU: Adelaide Academic Press, 2009.

Schou, Mogens. "Normothymotics, 'Mood-Normalizers: Are Lithium and the Imipramine Drugs Specific for Affective Disorders?'" *British Journal of Psychiatry* 109 (1963): 803–09.

Schou, Mogens. "The Rise of Lithium Treatment in the 1960s." In *The History of Psychopharmacology and the CINP, As Told in Autobiography*, Vol. 1, *The Rise of Psychopharmacology and the Story of CINP*, edited by Thomas A. Ban, David Healy, and Edward Shorter, 95–97. 2nd ed. Vienna: Collegium Internationale Neuro-Psychopharmacologicum, 2010.

Schou, Mogens. "Therapeutic and Toxic Properties of Lithium." In *Proceedings of the First International Congress of Neuropharmacology, Rome, September 1958*, edited by Philip Bradley, Pierre Deniker, and Corneille Raduoco-Thomas, 687–690. Amsterdam: Elsevier, 1959.

Schou, Mogens, N. Juel-Nielsen, Erik Strömgren, and H. Voldby. "The Treatment of Manic Psychoses by the Administration of Lithium Salts." *Journal of Neurology, Neurosurgery, and Psychiatry* 17, no. 4 (1954): 250–60.

Scull, Andrew. *Madhouse: A Tragic Tale of Megalomania and Modern Medicine*. New Haven, CT: Yale University Press, 2005.

Shorter, Edward. *A History of Psychiatry: From the Era of the Asylum to the Age of Prozac*. New York: John Wiley & Sons, 1997.

Strobusch, Alan D., and James W. Jefferson. "The Checkered History of Lithium in Medicine." *Pharmacy in History* 22, no. 2 (1980): 72–76. Accessed October 26, 2015, http://www.jstor.org/stable/i40048823.

Styron, William. *Darkness Visible: A Memoir of Madness*. New York: Random House, 1990.

Talbott, John H. "Use of Lithium Salts as a Substitute for Sodium Chloride." *Archives of Internal Medicine* 85, no. 1 (1950): 1–10.

Tondo, Leonardo, and Ross J. Baldessarini. "Antisuicidal Effects in Mood Disorders: Are They Unique to Lithium?" *Pharmacopsychiatry* 51 (April 2018): 177–88. doi: 10.1055/a-0596-7853.

Westmore, Ann. "The Many Faces of John Cade." In Johan Schioldann, *History of the Introduction of Lithium into Medicine and Psychiatry: Birth of Modern Psychopharmacology 1949*. Adelaide, AU: Adelaide Academic Press, 2009, Appendix 2, 310–11.

Westmore, Ann, and Greg de Moore. "The 'Mad Major' and His Idiosyncratic War: Linking Military Medicine and Lithium Therapy for Mania." *Health and History: Journal of the Australian & New Zealand Society for the History of Medicine* 15, no. 1 (2013): 11–37. Special issue: World War II and Medical Research in Australia.

Willis, Thomas. *Two Discourses Concerning the Soul of Brutes.* Translated by Samuel Pordage. London: Thomas Dring, 1683.

Yeragani, Vibram K., and Samuel Gershon. "Hammond and Lithium: Historical Update." *Biological Psychiatry* 21, no. 11 (1986): 1101–02.

Young, Allan H., and Judith M. Hammond. "Lithium in Mood Disorders: Increasing Evidence Base, Declining Use?" *British Journal of Psychiatry* 191, no. 6 (2007): 474–76.

INDEX